MY PREVENTION HEALTH ORGANIZER

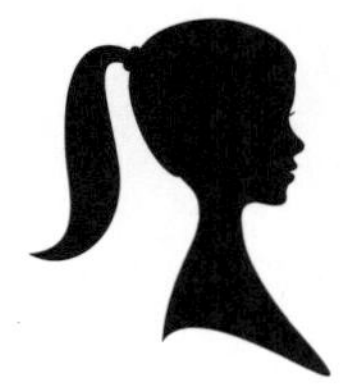

Take charge of your health with this essential planner and record-keeper

From the editors of Prevention.

RODALE

Library of Congress Cataloging-in-Publication Data
My prevention health organizer / by the editors of Prevention.
       p.   cm.
    ISBN-13 978-1-60529-356-1 hardcover
    ISBN-10 1-60529-356-3 hardcover
    1. Medicine, Popular.   2. Self-care, Health—Popular works.   I. Prevention (Emmaus, Pa.)
    RA776.5M95 2010
    613—dc22   2010015851

2   4   6   8   10   9   7   5   3   1   hardcover

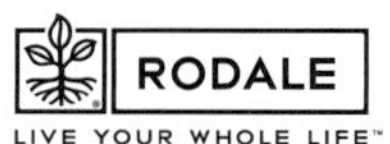

EVERYTHING WE DO AT *PREVENTION* is aimed at helping you live a healthy, satisfying life, which means preventing injury, illness, and other destructive influences from cramping your style. After all, preventing problems long before they arise is the best way to stay healthy, and the key to prevention is knowledge. Not just any kind of knowledge, either—you need thorough, detailed, organized information about yourself and your family to get a complete picture of what's going on inside you now and in the years to come.

My Prevention Health Organizer is designed to help you focus on the picture of your health. I hope you'll find it a fun, handy place to keep track of all that information everyone's been telling you to gather. It's organized into three parts:

• **IN PART 1, MY HEALTH RECORDS,** you'll be able to gather your complete health history and note the dates and results of your medical visits.

• **IN PART 2, MY CURRENT HEALTH,** you'll evaluate your weight, fitness, and other common measurements in relation to your goals.

• **IN PART 3, MY HEALTH JOURNAL,** you'll have space to monitor everything—from your hours of sleep to the foods you're eating to your mood—and observe how that affects your blood pressure, blood sugar levels, and other vital stats on a daily, weekly, monthly, and even yearly basis.

And, of course, you'll find plenty of reliable, actionable advice to help you understand what's going on with your body and to incorporate more good habits into your life.

Imagine how impressed your doctor will be when you show up to your next appointment armed with the answer to every question he has: what symptoms you've been experiencing, which tests your former doctor ran and what the results were, if you've ever had a bad reaction to a specific medication. You'll never have to search old files for your blood pressure measurements from 3 years ago or call Aunt Sally to see if anyone in the family has had diabetes. You'll know at a glance what tests you should be scheduling once you turn 25, or 32, or 53, and you'll have checklists to help you keep track of what you should be doing to care for yourself.

If knowledge is power, then with the help of *My Prevention Health Organizer* you're about to become an unstoppable force for improving and maintaining your health, now and for the rest of your life. And we'll be with you every step of the way.

—Liz Vaccariello

Editor-in-Chief, *Prevention* Magazine

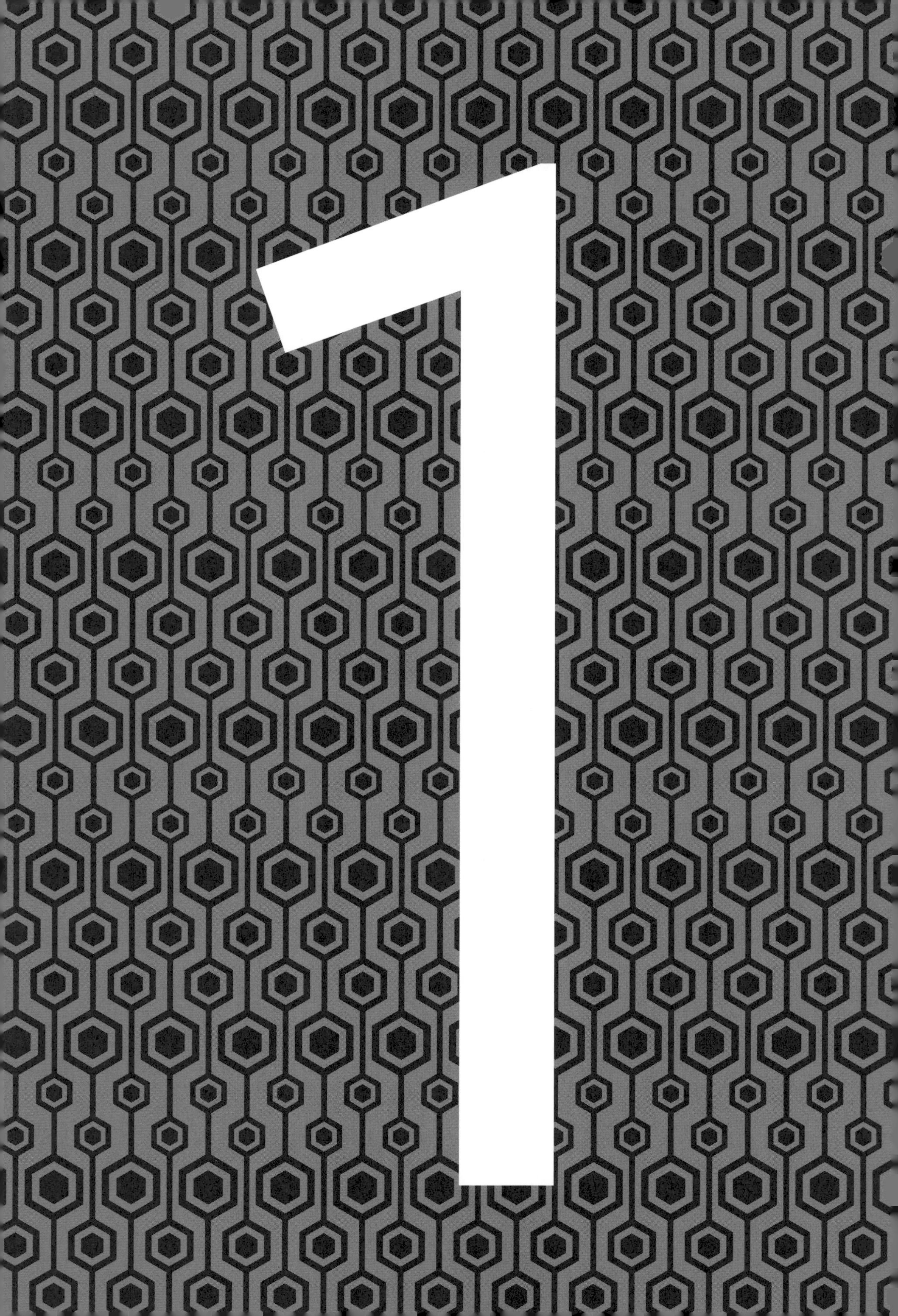

MY HEALTH RECORDS

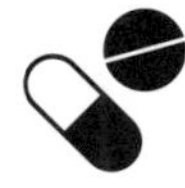
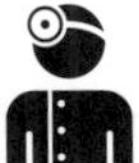
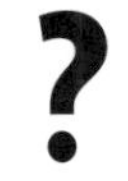
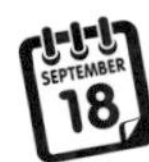
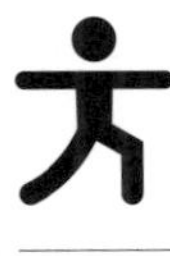
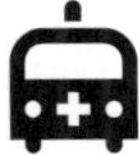

IN THIS ERA OF MANAGED CARE, it's important to be your own and your family's health advocate. To do that, you need information at your fingertips. In this section, we give you room to record your family's health history and track your symptoms, tests, and doctors' visits. You'll also find advice on when you need to go to the doctor (or emergency room) and how to make the most of your visits.

"Knowledge must come through action."

—SOPHOCLES

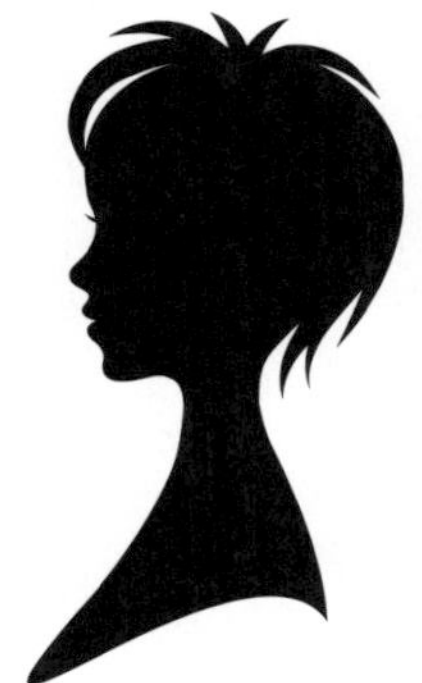

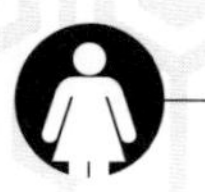

MY INFORMATION

NAME:

ADDRESS:

HOME PHONE NUMBER:

MOBILE PHONE NUMBER:

WORK PHONE: FAX NUMBER:

E-MAIL:

SOCIAL SECURITY NUMBER:

BASIC MEDICAL INFORMATION:

BLOOD TYPE:

ALLERGIES:

CHRONIC CONDITIONS:

CURRENT MEDICATIONS:

EMERGENCY CONTACTS

(IN ORDER OF PREFERENCE)

CONTACT 1 (IMMEDIATE FAMILY):

RELATION:

ADDRESS:

HOME PHONE NUMBER:

MOBILE PHONE NUMBER:

WORK PHONE NUMBER:

E-MAIL:

CONTACT 2:

RELATION:

ADDRESS:

HOME PHONE NUMBER:

MOBILE PHONE NUMBER:

WORK PHONE NUMBER:

E-MAIL:

CONTACT 3:

RELATION:

ADDRESS:

HOME PHONE NUMBER:

MOBILE PHONE NUMBER:

WORK PHONE NUMBER:

E-MAIL:

INSURANCE INFORMATION

EMPLOYER:

ADDRESS:

PHONE NUMBER:

FAX NUMBER:

E-MAIL ADDRESS/WEB SITE:

HR/BENEFITS CONTACT:

ADDRESS:

PHONE NUMBER

FAX NUMBER:

E-MAIL ADDRESS/WEB SITE:

PRIMARY INSURANCE COMPANY:

ADDRESS:

PHONE NUMBER:

FAX NUMBER:

E-MAIL ADDRESS/WEB SITE:

POLICYHOLDER:

DATE OF BIRTH:

EMPLOYER/GROUP:

SOCIAL SECURITY NUMBER:

PLAN TYPE:

POLICY NUMBER:

COPAYMENT:

COVERAGE LEVEL:

SECONDARY INSURANCE COMPANY:

ADDRESS:

PHONE NUMBER:

FAX NUMBER:

E-MAIL ADDRESS/WEB SITE:

PRESCRIPTION PLAN:

ADDRESS:

PHONE NUMBER:

FAX NUMBER:

E-MAIL ADDRESS/WEB SITE:

DEPENDENTS (IF APPLICABLE)

NAME:

RELATION:

SOCIAL SECURITY NUMBER:

DATE OF BIRTH:

NAME:

RELATION:

SOCIAL SECURITY NUMBER:

DATE OF BIRTH:

NAME:

RELATION:

SOCIAL SECURITY NUMBER:

DATE OF BIRTH:

MY HEALTH HISTORY

YOU ALREADY KNOW how important it is to share information about recent ailments and random symptoms with your doctor during your regular checkups. But did you know that a medication you took a few months ago might still affect your health today? Or that a pattern of illnesses over the last few years may give your doctor crucial clues as to the cause of a symptom you're experiencing now? The human body is a complex organism, and we can't always easily see how one aspect of our health may influence another.

Moreover, some diseases have a genetic component. For instance, if one of your parents was diagnosed with type 2 diabetes before age 50, your risk of developing the disease is 1 in 7; if your parent was diagnosed after age 50, your risk of getting diabetes is 1 in 13. Since a family history of type 2 diabetes is one of the strongest risk factors for getting the disease, but controllable environmental causes tend to trigger its onset, knowing your family health history and sharing it with your doctor can significantly improve your chances of preventing this type of diabetes. The same is true for many other conditions including heart disease and even certain types of cancer.

You've probably been asked to fill out forms requesting information on the prevalence of various conditions and medications in your personal and family history, but maybe you didn't know all the answers or have the details on hand. Completing this section and keeping it updated will allow you to attend your next appointment armed with all the facts necessary for you and your doctor to work together most effectively in keeping you at optimum health.

Personal Health Records

USING *My Prevention Health Organizer* will help you keep your most important health data in one place for easy reference, but it's also a good idea to keep copies of records from your doctors. To do this, you will need to request a copy of your health records from all of your health care providers, including your primary physician and any other specialists you have seen. Speak with your doctors' offices or medical records staff to find out if they can help you create personal health records (PHRs). You'll need to complete and return an authorization form, and most facilities will charge you for the cost of copying, including supplies, labor, and postage. Don't feel you have to gather everything at once. You can simply ask for recent records during your next office visit.

Once you've begun to compile your PHR, you'll need a way to store it. This can be as low tech as tossing some manila envelopes in a box (one per person) or as high tech as using an electronic program or a Web-based service. Some programs alert you via e-mail or text message if a family member has a medical emergency, if a drug you're taking is recalled, or when you need to schedule follow-up appointments. Some can upload information from medical devices (such as blood glucose monitors) directly to your files; others graph information so you can see health changes over time (www.prevention.com/healthtrackers offers such reports). And going electronic makes it a snap to search for names and results.

Whichever method you choose, make sure you also keep track of key information and store it someplace accessible. Make copies of the most vital stats (like allergies or serious health conditions) for your wallet and for the refrigerator (emergency medical technicians are trained to check there).

MY HEALTH HISTORY
worksheet

ALLERGIES:

DIETARY RESTRICTIONS:

Immunizations (DATE AND TYPE)

Vaccine	Date	Administered by	To be renewed
Tdap (Tetanus, diphtheria, acellular pertussis)	Last 1/12/2000	Dr. Smith	1/12/10

NOTES:

MEDICAL CONDITIONS:

TYPE:

DATE OF DIAGNOSIS: BY WHOM:

TESTS (AND RESULTS):

RELEVANT TREATMENTS *(hospitalizations, procedures, surgeries)*:

RELEVANT MEDICATIONS:

TYPE:

DATE OF DIAGNOSIS: BY WHOM:

TESTS (AND RESULTS):

RELEVANT TREATMENTS *(hospitalizations, procedures, surgeries)*:

RELEVANT MEDICATIONS:

TYPE:

DATE OF DIAGNOSIS: BY WHOM:

TESTS (AND RESULTS):

RELEVANT TREATMENTS *(hospitalizations, procedures, surgeries)*:

RELEVANT MEDICATIONS:

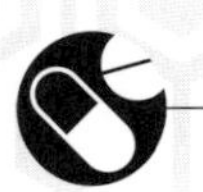

MY MEDICATIONS AND PRESCRIPTIONS

T'S IMPORTANT THAT YOU ALWAYS follow dosing instructions exactly. They ensure that your body will process the medication in a way that will be helpful to you. For example, medication taken on an empty stomach will be processed much differently by your body than will medication taken on a full stomach. Not following the directions could prevent the medication from doing its job, or it could even cause serious health problems. So read those instructions and follow them carefully!

Individuals process drugs differently, based on a range of factors including age, gender, weight, diet, health history, racial/ethnic background, and individual genetics. Medication dosages and side effects are determined based on studies of the broader population and may not be accurate for every individual. Be sure to closely monitor any effects you experience as a result of the medications you're prescribed, and speak with your doctor immediately about any problems. Also, be open with your doctor about your diet and lifestyle, including your use of cigarettes or consumption of alcohol, vitamins, herbal supplements, and any other substances, even illegal ones—these will all affect the ways in which your body responds to medications.

Date prescribed	Medication name	Dose(s)	Time(s)	Instructions	Effects (positive & negative)	Doctor name/phone	Pharmacy name/phone
11/2/09	Albuterol	1 puff	Morning	Breathe out fully before inhaling	Some lightheadedness w/2 puffs	Dr. Walker 655-555-1212	Corner Pharmacy 655-555-1414
		2 puffs	As needed	Take immediately when needed	Breathing improves w/in 1–2 minutes		

QUESTIONS FOR DOCTOR: ____

____

MY SIBLINGS' HEALTH HISTORY
worksheet

MY SIBLING: _______________________________ BIRTHDATE: _______________

MEDICAL CONDITIONS *(type, date of diagnosis, and age at time of diagnosis):*

____

____

OPERATIONS/PROCEDURES *(type, date, and age at time of procedure):*

____

____

ALLERGIES:

____

____

OTHER:

____

MY SIBLING: _______________________________ BIRTHDATE: _______________

MEDICAL CONDITIONS *(type, date of diagnosis, and age at time of diagnosis):*

____

____

OPERATIONS/PROCEDURES *(type, date, and age at time of procedure):*

____

____

ALLERGIES:

____

____

OTHER:

____

MY MOTHER'S
FAMILY HEALTH HISTORY
worksheet

MOTHER: BIRTHDATE:

MEDICAL CONDITIONS *(type, date of diagnosis, and age at time of diagnosis):*

OPERATIONS/PROCEDURES *(type, date, and age at time of procedure):*

ALLERGIES:

MATERNAL GRANDMOTHER: BIRTHDATE:

MEDICAL CONDITIONS *(type, date of diagnosis, and age at time of diagnosis):*

OPERATIONS/PROCEDURES *(type, date, and age at time of procedure):*

ALLERGIES:

MATERNAL GRANDFATHER: BIRTHDATE:

MEDICAL CONDITIONS *(type, date of diagnosis, and age at time of diagnosis):*

OPERATIONS/PROCEDURES *(type, date, and age at time of procedure)*:

ALLERGIES:

MOTHER'S SIBLING: BIRTHDATE:

MEDICAL CONDITIONS *(type, date of diagnosis, and age at time of diagnosis)*:

OPERATIONS/PROCEDURES *(type, date, and age at time of procedure)*:

ALLERGIES:

MOTHER'S SIBLING: BIRTHDATE:

MEDICAL CONDITIONS *(type, date of diagnosis, and age at time of diagnosis)*:

OPERATIONS/PROCEDURES *(type, date, and age at time of procedure)*:

ALLERGIES:

OTHER NOTES:

MY FATHER'S
FAMILY HEALTH HISTORY
worksheet

FATHER: _______________________ BIRTHDATE: _______________________

MEDICAL CONDITIONS *(type, date of diagnosis, and age at time of diagnosis):* _______________________

____

____

OPERATIONS/PROCEDURES *(type, date, and age at time of procedure):* _______________________

____

____

ALLERGIES: _______________________

____

____

PATERNAL GRANDMOTHER: _______________________ BIRTHDATE: _______________________

MEDICAL CONDITIONS *(type, date of diagnosis, and age at time of diagnosis):* _______________________

____

____

OPERATIONS/PROCEDURES *(type, date, and age at time of procedure):* _______________________

____

____

ALLERGIES: _______________________

____

PATERNAL GRANDFATHER: _______________________ BIRTHDATE: _______________________

MEDICAL CONDITIONS *(type, date of diagnosis, and age at time of diagnosis):* _______________________

____

____

OPERATIONS/PROCEDURES *(type, date, and age at time of procedure):*

ALLERGIES:

FATHER'S SIBLING: BIRTHDATE:

MEDICAL CONDITIONS *(type, date of diagnosis, and age at time of diagnosis):*

OPERATIONS/PROCEDURES *(type, date, and age at time of procedure):*

ALLERGIES:

FATHER'S SIBLING: BIRTHDATE:

MEDICAL CONDITIONS *(type, date of diagnosis, and age at time of diagnosis):*

OPERATIONS/PROCEDURES *(type, date, and age at time of procedure):*

ALLERGIES:

OTHER NOTES:

MY SPOUSE'S HEALTH HISTORY
worksheet

While this organizer is designed to hold your health information, not your whole family's, we thought you might find this a convenient place to note just the basics of your spouse's health history so that it's handy in case of an emergency. Feel free to photocopy this page if you prefer to record more detail.

MEDICAL CONDITIONS *(type, date, and age at time of diagnosis):*

OPERATIONS/PROCEDURES *(type, date, and age at time of procedure):*

ALLERGIES:

Immunizations:

Vaccine	Date	Administered by	To be renewed

Past Medications:

Medication name	Dose(s)/Times(s)	Instructions	Effects

MY CHILDREN'S HEALTH HISTORY
worksheet

While this organizer is designed to hold your health information, not your whole family's, we thought you might find this a convenient place to note just the basics of your children's health history so that it's handy in case of an emergency. Feel free to photocopy this page if you prefer to record more detail.

MEDICAL CONDITIONS *(type, date, and age at time of diagnosis):*

____

____

OPERATIONS/PROCEDURES *(type, date, and age at time of procedure):*

____

____

ALLERGIES:

____

____

Immunizations:

Vaccine	Date	Administered by	To be renewed

Past Medications:

Medication name	Dose(s)/Times(s)	Instructions	Effects

MY DOCTORS

GENERAL PRACTITIONER'S NAME:

ADDRESS:

PHONE NUMBER: E-MAIL ADDRESS/WEB SITE:

EMERGENCY NUMBER: FAX NUMBER:

AFFILIATED HOSPITALS:

ALTERNATE OFFICE LOCATIONS:

DENTIST'S NAME:

ADDRESS:

PHONE NUMBER: E-MAIL ADDRESS/WEB SITE:

EMERGENCY NUMBER: FAX NUMBER:

AFFILIATED HOSPITALS:

ALTERNATE OFFICE LOCATIONS:

OBSTETRICIAN/GYNECOLOGIST'S NAME:

ADDRESS:

PHONE NUMBER: E-MAIL ADDRESS/WEB SITE:

EMERGENCY NUMBER: FAX NUMBER:

AFFILIATED HOSPITALS:

ALTERNATE OFFICE LOCATIONS:

OTHER SPECIALIST'S NAME:

ADDRESS:

PHONE NUMBER: E-MAIL ADDRESS/WEB SITE:

EMERGENCY NUMBER: FAX NUMBER:

AFFILIATED HOSPITALS:

ALTERNATE OFFICE LOCATIONS:

OTHER SPECIALIST'S NAME:

ADDRESS:

PHONE NUMBER: E-MAIL ADDRESS/WEB SITE:

EMERGENCY NUMBER: FAX NUMBER:

AFFILIATED HOSPITALS:

ALTERNATE OFFICE LOCATIONS:

OTHER SPECIALIST'S NAME:

ADDRESS:

PHONE NUMBER: E-MAIL ADDRESS/WEB SITE:

EMERGENCY NUMBER: FAX NUMBER:

AFFILIATED HOSPITALS:

ALTERNATE OFFICE LOCATIONS:

MAKE THE MOST OF YOUR DOCTOR'S VISIT

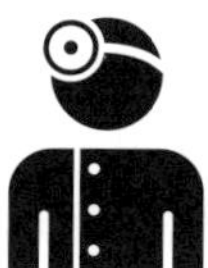

IT HAPPENS OFTEN ENOUGH that doctors have a nickname for it: "the doorknob complaint." You know, that last little question you blurt out just as your doctor is saying good-bye and opening the door? Maybe you left this important health question for the very last minute because you were too embarrassed to bring it up sooner. Maybe you started to address it, but the doctor's interruption took you off in another direction. Or maybe you had other issues you wanted to cover first, and this one just got shoved to the end of the list. Whatever the reason for your delay, "doorknob complaints" can pose a problem for you and your doctor because he or she may not have much time or focus left for this concern if you wait until they're leaving. "They can come back and re-engage, but they've already signaled to you that they have time pressure, and it's not going to be the same kind of conversation as before the hand touched the doorknob," says Melissa Piasecki, MD, professor of psychiatry at the University of Nevada and author of a handbook for doctors to improve their patient communication skills. "I think everyone would acknowledge that it's not ideal for something important to come up after the doorknob is touched." We at *Prevention* want to make sure that your health concerns get the attention they deserve, so we've developed this section to help you ensure that from now on your visits go smoothly and that you get a satisfactory answer to all your questions. If these strategies still don't get you the answers you need, don't hesitate to get a second opinion.

☐ **KNOW YOUR SYMPTOMS.** Get in the habit of recording when a symptom begins as well as other details such as how frequently it occurs, if it's increased or lessened, where it's happening in your body, what it feels like, if there is any pain, and what kind of pain you feel. Use the My Symptom Tracker beginning on page 26 to record as many details about your symptoms as possible, and don't forget to take your Health Organizer with you to your next appointment. It's important to discuss your symptoms with your doctor before they become severe or urgent, so prioritize, but don't be afraid to bring something up. Also, never postpone seeing your doctor if you have symptoms that cause you severe pain or if you notice an increase in frequency of pain.

☐ **KNOW WHAT YOU WANT TO DISCUSS.** During your appointment, you and your doctor will likely each have a different list of things you want to address. You may have symptoms to ask about, need a prescription refill, or want to schedule a test you've heard recommended for your age group (the My Health Decade by Decade section includes handy checklists of such recommendations). Your doctor has a limited amount of time to listen to your symptoms, prescribe the right tests or treatments, and make sure you leave satisfied. You'll want to go prepared to cover everything in an organized, time-efficient way. That means prioritizing your list—review your Symptom Tracker, and group symptoms you think might be related, such as a sore throat and a cough. Then number these groups according to what's most important or what you're most concerned about. Finally, make a clean copy of the list in order of priority to give to your doctor. He or she may spot something at #8 that has more importance than you're aware of. "Doctors want information, but they want specific information presented in specific ways. The more organized the person is when they come in, the smoother and more complete the information transfer's going to be," Dr. Piasecki says.

☐ **TAKE COPIES OF VITAL INFORMATION.** The more complete a picture your doctor can get of your health and daily habits, the better he or she will be able to understand your complaints. You'll want to take records of your recent blood pressure, blood sugar, weight changes, and anything else pertinent to your chronic health problems (your doctor may have some of these if he or she is your primary care physician). You'll also want to have a list of any medications, vitamins, and supplements you've taken recently. Be prepared to discuss any significant changes in habit, such as a new diet or exercise regimen. And take this organizer—the My Current Health and My Health Journal sections are the perfect places to keep track of this information.

☐ **DON'T BE AFRAID OF YOUR DOCTOR.** Even the nicest physicians can sometimes come across as brusque, but that's just because health care is a bit of a whirlwind. Your doctor may be rushing from appointment to appointment, not to mention unscheduled sick visits and emergencies. By helping set the agenda and expressing your concerns in an organized way, you're more likely to have a satisfying visit. However, if your doctor is moving fast and you aren't getting to something that's important to you, don't be afraid to interrupt. Be firm without being pushy and you'll be more likely to get the answers you need.

☐ **BE READY TO WATCH AND WAIT.** Not every ache or bump you detect will point to a serious underlying illness. Sometimes a symptom is just a minor, fleeting ailment or may be treatable with simple self-care or over-the-counter remedies. Your doctor may prescribe tests or ask you to keep an eye on it, with instructions to call if anything changes for the worse. If you've given your doctor a complete medical history and a thorough description of your symptoms and they don't believe your problem is serious at this time, trust their judgment. That's why you went to that doctor in the first place, isn't it?

☐ **FOLLOW YOUR DOCTOR'S INSTRUCTIONS.** Your doctor may tell you to call in a week if you're still having headaches, or you may receive a prescription. They may ask you to measure a swollen knee or chart your energy levels. Whatever the instructions, it's critically important that you follow the doctor's orders. It's also important to ask what your next step should be—how soon will you see an improvement after starting your medication, or what side effects should you be alert for? Listen to the answers. Good follow-through will ensure that your doctor's care continues even after you leave the office and that you'll be able to catch any adverse changes before they become a problem. If you follow instructions and the outcome isn't as your doctor described, you'll know to call and make another appointment or receive new instructions.

> **"Every patient carries his or her own doctor inside."**
>
> —ALBERT SCHWEITZER

QUESTIONS TO ASK YOUR DOCTOR

USE THIS SECTION as a place to record questions you want to have answered at your next appointment. In addition to any symptoms you may want to ask about, be sure to include important follow-up questions. These will vary depending on what your doctor instructs you to do, but some questions you might want to ask include:

Can I make lifestyle changes or start a new fitness regime to treat this symptom initially, or do you recommend medication?

Would physical therapy be useful for treating this condition?

I've heard that people my age should get tested for [X]. What do you think?

Are there any activities, foods, or supplements you recommend I avoid or begin using to maintain my health?

Are there any new vaccines or treatments you think I should look into?

Is surgery an option (and is it the only one)?

Can you recommend a specialist I should see to deal with this health issue?

IF YOU'RE PRESCRIBED MEDICATION, MAKE SURE YOU ASK:

Do I need to take this medication with food or at a certain time of day?

How often do I need to take this and for how long?

What do I do if I forget a dose?

Are there any side effects I should particularly watch out for?

Are there any foods, supplements, or other medications I should avoid while I take this?

When should I expect to see relief?

ADDITIONAL QUESTIONS:

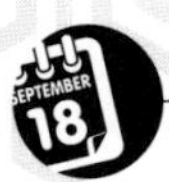

MY APPOINTMENTS

Year:

PRIMARY CARE PROVIDER:

CHECKUP/WELL VISIT DATE:

NOTES:

SICK VISIT DATE:

NOTES:

SICK VISIT DATE:

NOTES:

DENTIST:

CHECKUP/WELL VISIT DATE:

NOTES:

CHECKUP/WELL VISIT DATE:

NOTES:

SICK VISIT DATE:

NOTES:

SICK VISIT DATE:

NOTES:

OBSTETRICIAN/GYNECOLOGIST:

CHECKUP/WELL VISIT DATE:

NOTES:

SICK VISIT DATE:

NOTES:

SICK VISIT DATE:

NOTES:

OTHER SPECIALIST:

VISIT DATE:

NOTES:

OTHER SPECIALIST:

VISIT DATE:

NOTES:

OTHER SPECIALIST:

VISIT DATE:

NOTES:

OTHER SPECIALIST:

VISIT DATE:

NOTES:

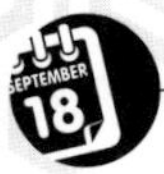

MY APPOINTMENTS

Year:

PRIMARY CARE PROVIDER:

CHECKUP/WELL VISIT DATE:

NOTES:

SICK VISIT DATE:

NOTES:

SICK VISIT DATE:

NOTES:

DENTIST:

CHECKUP/WELL VISIT DATE:

NOTES:

CHECKUP/WELL VISIT DATE:

NOTES:

SICK VISIT DATE:

NOTES:

SICK VISIT DATE:

NOTES:

OBSTETRICIAN/GYNECOLOGIST:

CHECKUP/WELL VISIT DATE:

NOTES:

SICK VISIT DATE:

NOTES:

SICK VISIT DATE:

NOTES:

OTHER SPECIALIST:

VISIT DATE:

NOTES:

OTHER SPECIALIST:

VISIT DATE:

NOTES:

OTHER SPECIALIST:

VISIT DATE:

NOTES:

OTHER SPECIALIST:

VISIT DATE:

NOTES:

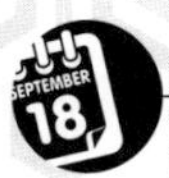

MY APPOINTMENTS

Year:

PRIMARY CARE PROVIDER:

CHECKUP/WELL VISIT DATE:

NOTES:

SICK VISIT DATE:

NOTES:

SICK VISIT DATE:

NOTES:

DENTIST:

CHECKUP/WELL VISIT DATE:

NOTES:

CHECKUP/WELL VISIT DATE:

NOTES:

SICK VISIT DATE:

NOTES:

SICK VISIT DATE:

NOTES:

OBSTETRICIAN/GYNECOLOGIST:

CHECKUP/WELL VISIT DATE:

NOTES:

SICK VISIT DATE:

NOTES:

SICK VISIT DATE:

NOTES:

OTHER SPECIALIST:

VISIT DATE:

NOTES:

OTHER SPECIALIST:

VISIT DATE:

NOTES:

OTHER SPECIALIST:

VISIT DATE:

NOTES:

OTHER SPECIALIST:

VISIT DATE:

NOTES:

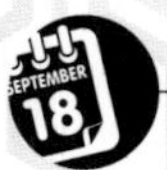

MY APPOINTMENTS

Year:

PRIMARY CARE PROVIDER:

CHECKUP/WELL VISIT DATE:

NOTES:

SICK VISIT DATE:

NOTES:

SICK VISIT DATE:

NOTES:

DENTIST:

CHECKUP/WELL VISIT DATE:

NOTES:

CHECKUP/WELL VISIT DATE:

NOTES:

SICK VISIT DATE:

NOTES:

SICK VISIT DATE:

NOTES:

OBSTETRICIAN/GYNECOLOGIST:

CHECKUP/WELL VISIT DATE:

NOTES:

SICK VISIT DATE:

NOTES:

SICK VISIT DATE:

NOTES:

OTHER SPECIALIST:

VISIT DATE:

NOTES:

OTHER SPECIALIST:

VISIT DATE:

NOTES:

OTHER SPECIALIST:

VISIT DATE:

NOTES:

OTHER SPECIALIST:

VISIT DATE:

NOTES:

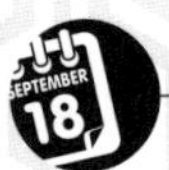

MY APPOINTMENTS

Year:

PRIMARY CARE PROVIDER:

CHECKUP/WELL VISIT DATE:

NOTES:

SICK VISIT DATE:

NOTES:

SICK VISIT DATE:

NOTES:

DENTIST:

CHECKUP/WELL VISIT DATE:

NOTES:

CHECKUP/WELL VISIT DATE:

NOTES:

SICK VISIT DATE:

NOTES:

SICK VISIT DATE:

NOTES:

OBSTETRICIAN/GYNECOLOGIST:

CHECKUP/WELL VISIT DATE:

NOTES:

SICK VISIT DATE:

NOTES:

SICK VISIT DATE:

NOTES:

OTHER SPECIALIST:

VISIT DATE:

NOTES:

OTHER SPECIALIST:

VISIT DATE:

NOTES:

OTHER SPECIALIST:

VISIT DATE:

NOTES:

OTHER SPECIALIST:

VISIT DATE:

NOTES:

MY SYMPTOM TRACKER

MINOR ACHES AND PAINS or a little itch here and there is common fare for this complicated, ever-changing vehicle we call the human body. And as we age, the frequency with which we experience these mild annoyances can increase. But do you know which to ignore and which should prompt you to seek medical attention? Preventative care is the number one way to avoid developing serious threats to your health. Use this section to keep track of any little messages your body might be sending you, paying particular attention to anything that occurs regularly, with increasing frequency, or with increasing severity over time. Be as specific as you can in describing the problem as well as noting where and when it occurs so that you can pass your doctor all the information he or she needs to choose an appropriate course of action.

WHOLE-BODY SYMPTOMS

- Appetite loss
- Body odor
- Dizziness/light-headedness
- Excessive thirst
- Fatigue
- Fever
- Insomnia
- Sweating
- Weight gain
- Weight loss

PAIN SYMPTOMS

- General pain
- Headache
- Joint stiffness
- Joint pain
- Muscle aches
- Muscle cramping

MIND AND MOOD SYMPTOMS

- Anxiety
- Confusion
- Depression
- Forgetfulness
- Mood swings
- Poor concentration

EYE/VISION SYMPTOMS

- Blurred vision
- Eye discharge
- Dry eyes
- Red eyes

EAR SYMPTOMS

- Earache
- Ear discharge
- Difficulty hearing
- Ringing in the ears

NASAL/RESPIRATORY SYMPTOMS

- Congestion
- Nosebleeds
- Rapid breathing
- Runny nose
- Sneezing
- Wheezing/shortness of breath

MOUTH SYMPTOMS

- Bad breath (halitosis)
- Bleeding gums
- Canker sores
- Cold sores
- Dry mouth
- Tooth pain

THROAT SYMPTOMS

- Cough
- Hoarseness
- Sore throat

CARDIOVASCULAR SYMPTOMS

- Chest pain
- Irregular heartbeat
- Rapid heartbeat

DIGESTIVE SYMPTOMS

- Abdominal pain
- Black or bloody stool
- Bloating
- Constipation
- Diarrhea
- Gas
- Heartburn
- Indigestion
- Nausea/vomiting
- Stomach pain

URINARY SYMPTOMS

- Blood in urine
- Burning upon urination
- Difficulty urinating
- Incontinence
- Frequent urination

SKIN AND HAIR SYMPTOMS

- Blisters
- Bruising
- Excessive hair growth
- Hair loss
- Itching
- Pimples
- Moles
- Rash
- Redness
- Scaling

SEXUAL/REPRODUCTIVE SYMPTOMS—WOMEN

- Breast pain
- Cramping
- Genital warts
- Hot flashes
- Low libido
- Vaginal bleeding
- Vaginal discharge
- Vaginal itching

SEXUAL/REPRODUCTIVE SYMPTOMS—MEN

- Blood in semen
- Erectile dysfunction
- Premature ejaculation
- Testicular swelling or pain

Symptom Tracker

Date	Time	Symptoms	Observation
11/19/09	Around 1 p.m., right after lunch	Simultaneously felt gassy and slightly nauseous	Got steadily worse through the afternoon

Symptom Tracker

Date	Time	Symptoms	Observation

KNOW THE SIGNS OF AN EMERGENCY

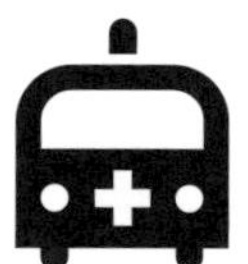 **SOMETIMES SYMPTOMS** point to a life-threatening emergency or a disease that should be treated immediately. If you notice any of the following symptoms, call your doctor immediately, or possibly call 911 or other emergency medical services. (A handy tear-sheet version of this list appears at the back of this organizer.)

☐ **CHEST PAIN.** It could just be gas, an involuntary muscle spasm, or something as serious as a heart attack. Usually, a heart attack will cause pain or an uncomfortable pressure or squeezing sensation that starts in the center of your chest and may spread to your arms, back, neck, or jaw. In addition to the pain, you may feel out of breath, nauseous, and light-headed, and you may break out into a cold sweat. Women often experience more discomfort, pressure, or tightness in their chests and the other above-mentioned symptoms than actual pain. If you think you're having a heart attack, call 911 immediately.

☐ **SHORTNESS OF BREATH.** In addition to a wide variety of conditions such as asthma and lung disease, difficulty breathing can also be a symptom of anaphylactic shock. This is a full-body allergic reaction that can be life-threatening. Other symptoms include confusion, light-headedness, hives, heart palpitations, and nausea. It can result from insect stings, certain foods, medications, or other factors that trigger allergic reactions—if you experience trouble breathing following any of these events, call 911. Otherwise, call your doctor for advice.

☐ **LOSS OF CONSCIOUSNESS.** There are dozens of reasons a person might lose consciousness, many of them relatively harmless. However, if you pass out for an extended period of time or if your loss of consciousness is accompanied by confusion, deep and rapid breathing, seizures, and skin that is hot, dry, and flushed after exposure to hot weather, call 911. You may be suffering from heatstroke, an extreme form of heat exhaustion that can cause coma, brain damage, and even death.

☐ **BLOODY STOOL.** If you notice bleeding during a bowel movement, it could be due to a variety of causes anywhere along your digestive system. Bloody stool may appear black and tarry or more burgundy or bright red depending on where it's coming from. Call your doctor. If accompanied by weakness, call 911.

☐ **UNCONTROLLABLE BLEEDING.** If you have a bloody nose that just won't stop or are bleeding from the ears, vomiting blood, or have a minor injury that won't clot, call 911. The body's ability to form blood clots can be affected by a variety of illnesses, but regardless of cause, your body cannot withstand the loss of too much blood.

☐ **NUMBNESS OR WEAKNESS.** If your face, arm, or leg gets numb or weak—particularly if it's on one side of your body—call 911 or ask someone to do it for you. This could be a sign of a stroke, which is caused by a blockage of blood flow or bleeding in the brain.

☐ **SUDDEN LOSS OF ABILITIES.** If you realize you can't walk, see, or speak properly or you're having trouble thinking or understanding what other people are saying, call 911 or have someone do it for you. These could also be signs of a stroke.

☐ **UNUSUAL HEADACHES.** We all get headaches, but some are more serious than others. Call 911 if you have a sudden, severe headache, especially if you've suffered a head injury or if the headache is accompanied by a stiff neck, fever, rash, difficulty concentrating, or seizures. If you are experiencing less severe headaches and have not recently suffered a head injury or are having seizures, call your doctor first. Serious causes of these can include bleeding in the brain, stroke, meningitis, or a brain tumor.

☐ **LUMPS OR THICKENED SPOTS.** If you can feel a lump or raised spot in your body, you'll want your doctor to examine it. A lump could be an early cancer, but there are also many other issues that cause lumps and bumps in the body.

☐ **BLEEDING OR UNUSUAL DISCHARGE.** Unexpected blood or other fluid can be a sign of serious illnesses, even cancer. This includes bloody phlegm (material you cough up); blood in the urine; blood or discharge from the nipple; bloody vomit; or unusual vaginal bleeding. Make an appointment with your doctor if you notice any of these issues.

☐ **HARMFUL THOUGHTS.** Depression is more common than most people think, but there's a big difference between feeling blue and feeling suicidal. Sometimes depression can be an indicator of other mental illnesses as well. If you're thinking about hurting yourself or someone else, call your doctor or suicide hotline right away.

☐ **HEARING VOICES OR SEEING THINGS.** Hallucinations can be caused by serious physical conditions and medications as well as urgent mental health issues. Call your doctor immediately if you're experiencing these symptoms.

☐ **INTENSE, UNEXPLAINABLE FEAR.** This is a symptom of a panic attack, often accompanied by sweating, pounding heart, shortness of breath, and shaking. Panic attacks can severely affect your life, but they're treatable. Though your fear may cause you to think you need emergency help, call your doctor first.

~~~~~~

> **"In the field of observation, chance favors the prepared mind."**
>
> —LOUIS PASTEUR
~~~~~~

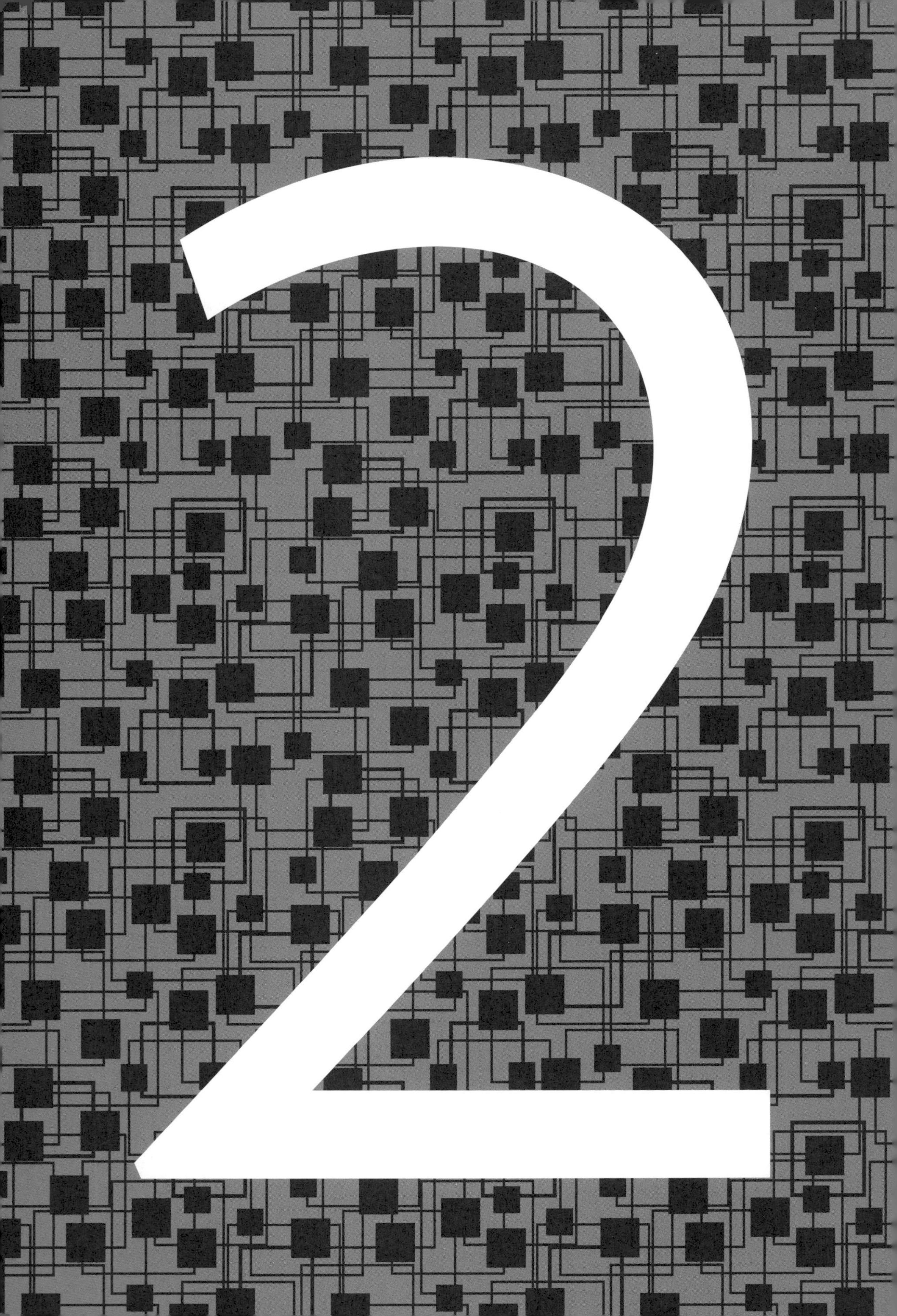

MY CURRENT HEALTH

WHATEVER YOUR ULTIMATE GOALS, you need to know your current status. In this section, we give you a primer on common tests and measurements to help you evaluate your fitness and overall health and set realistic weight loss and other health goals. And, since your needs change as you age, you'll find a decade-by-decade guide to help you keep current with important diagnostic tests, deal with essential health issues at every stage of your life, and make small changes that will have a big impact on your lifelong health and well-being.

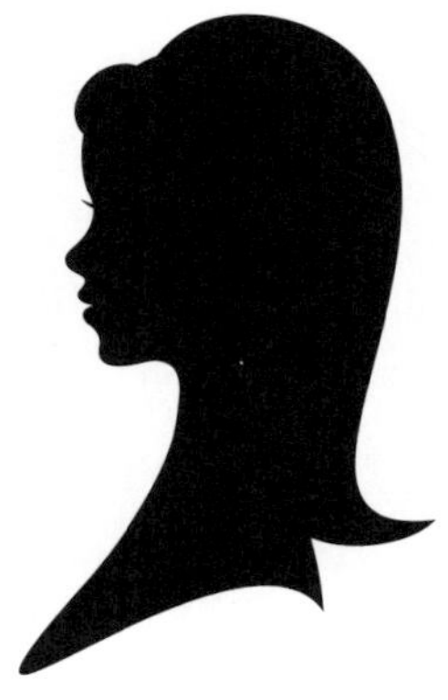

> **"Keeping your body healthy is an expression of gratitude to the whole cosmos."**
>
> —THICH NHAT HANH

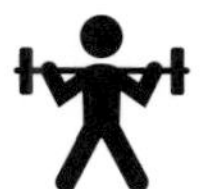  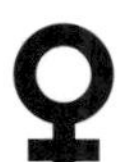 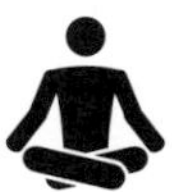 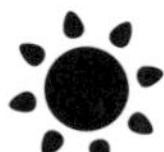 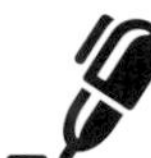

MY HEALTH MEASURES

Common Health Measures

WHETHER YOU WANT TO INCREASE your endurance, trim your tummy, lower your blood pressure, or just feel healthier, it's important to know where you're starting and track your progress. What follows is a list of the most common health measures—usually taken by your doctor at your annual checkup—that form a good basic picture of your overall health status. Problems with these measures are often the first indicators of important health issues that require attention. If your annual visit reveals some abnormality, your doctor may ask you to come in for follow-up testing or to take the measures yourself more frequently.

We encourage you to repeat these measurements (along with some basic fitness tests—see page 48) regularly. How often you measure will depend on your goals and the nature of the measurement—for example, your fitness stats will change quickly if you're exercising frequently, while cholesterol levels might take a bit longer to respond. Some measures you won't be able to take yourself, but you can obtain them easily at drugstores, clinics, and your doctor's office (we'll tell you which and where). Mark your starting measures in this section and then use My Yearly Health Tracker to monitor those your doctor asks you to track. Seeing the progress you're making will help you stay motivated to keep working toward your goal!

☐ **WEIGHT AND BMI**: Check your body mass index (BMI) using the chart on page 47. The BMI scale gives a picture of your total body fat in proportion to your overall body mass. This measure is widely used as a general assessment of health risks associated with weight. It is a more accurate indication of total body fat than weight alone. You're considered overweight if your BMI is between 25 and 29 and obese if your BMI is 30 or more. A low BMI is also considered unhealthy. Keep in mind that even BMI is far from a perfect measurement. Be sure to monitor several indicators such as your waist circumference and fitness test results, and determine your overall level of health based on all of them as opposed to focusing too much on just your weight and BMI.

Healthy level: between 18.5 and 25

How often: Annually if within healthy ranges, monthly or weekly if you are trying to lose or gain weight to reach healthy levels.

☐ **WAIST CIRCUMFERENCE**: Waist circumference is the distance around your natural waist, just above the navel. It helps determine the level of abdominal fat, which is associated with an increased risk of heart disease when compared with fat deposits in other areas of the body. An unhealthy waist circumference measurement can indicate a heightened risk of diabetes, hypertension, and cardiovascular disease. This measurement should be examined in connection with your BMI (see above) for a clearer picture of your overall health.

Healthy level: 35 inches for women; 40 inches for men

How often: Annually if within healthy ranges, monthly or weekly if you are trying to lose or gain weight to reach healthy levels.

☐ **BLOOD PRESSURE:** The top number in a blood pressure (BP) reading, called the systolic pressure, is the amount of force or pressure exerted against the arteries during each heartbeat. The lower or diastolic number represents the amount of pressure in the arteries between heartbeats. High blood pressure forces the heart to work harder to pump blood throughout the body, and it also contributes to hardening of the arteries and the possibility of heart failure. Any medical professional can take this measure for you, and many drugstores provide blood pressure machines for public use for the cost of a few quarters. However, if you are instructed to keep a close eye on your BP, invest in your own machine, available at many drugstores and online.

Healthy level: Below 120/80 mmHg

How often: Every 2 years, more frequently following your doctor's instruction if it's high.

☐ **HIGH DENSITY LIPOPROTEIN (HDL) CHOLESTEROL:** This "good" cholesterol ferries "bad" (LDL) cholesterol out of your blood, keeping it from building up in your arteries and thus protecting your heart. Because HDL protects you against heart disease, higher levels are good. A less-than-healthy level of HDL cholesterol can be a major risk factor for heart disease. Unfortunately, you'll need blood drawn to get this measure, so you can't do it yourself. Any doctor's office, hospital, or clinic can run this test—called a blood lipid profile—for you. You'll often find special free or low-cost cholesterol test events at your local hospital or university health clinic.

Healthy level: 50+ mg/dL for women; 40+ mg/dL for men. **Optimal level:** 60 mg/dL.

How often: Every 5 years starting at age 20; every 4 months if results are abnormal.

☐ **LOW DENSITY LIPOPROTEIN (LDL) CHOLESTEROL:** LDL is considered "bad" cholesterol because it leads to a buildup of plaque on your artery walls, which increases the likelihood of suffering a heart attack or stroke. As with HDL cholesterol, you'll need blood drawn to get this measure, so you can't do it yourself. Any doctor's office, hospital, or clinic can run the blood lipid profile for you. You'll often find special free or low-cost cholesterol test events at your local hospital or university health clinic.

Healthy level: Less than 129 mg/dL. **Optimal level:** Less than 100 mg/dL.

How often: Every 5 years starting at age 20; every 4 months if results are abnormal.

☐ **TRIGLYCERIDES:** Triglycerides are the main form of fat in the body—simply put, they are fat molecules in the bloodstream. Risk factors from a high triglyceride level can be hard to determine because it tends to coexist with high cholesterol and high blood pressure, but it does appear to increase risk of heart disease, metabolic syndrome, and diabetes. This is usually done as part of your blood lipid profile, a test you will have done at your doctor's office, a clinic, or a lab.

Healthy level: Less than 150 mg/dL

How often: Every 5 years starting at age 20; every 4 months if results are abnormal.

☐ **BLOOD SUGAR (FASTING BLOOD GLUCOSE LEVEL):** While it's normal for blood sugar to increase after a meal, levels that remain high over time can result in damage to eyes, kidneys, nerves, and blood vessels, and can lead to diabetes and metabolic syndrome. There are several types of blood sugar tests, but the fasting blood glucose level is the most commonly measured for early indications of blood sugar–related problems. It reveals excess amounts of glucose in the blood when no food has recently been introduced (and thus couldn't be the cause). This measure requires that you have blood drawn after abstaining from food for at least 12 hours (first thing in the morning works for most people). See your doctor about getting tested.

Healthy level (after fasting): 70 to 99 mg/dL. **Optimal level:** 70 to 90 mg/dL.

How often: Immediately if you're at high risk for diabetes, and every 3 years. If you are a diabetic, you'll need to measure more frequently according to your doctor's instructions.

Don't-Sweat-It Guide to Health

 HAVE TROUBLE keeping track of all the right foods you're supposed to eat or finding the time for the exercise you're supposed to be getting? Don't sweat it! Follow these recommendations and find the good-enough route to a longer, healthier life.

→ Fruits and Vegetables
Gold Standard: up to nine servings of fruits and vegetables a day
Good Enough: five a day
Experts have found that five servings provide antioxidants that reduce risk of heart disease and cancer. You can work up to five or more servings more easily than you think. For one serving, choose 15 grapes, 6 strawberries, 1 cup of orange or other fruit juice, 10 baby carrots, 1 cup of greens, or one large piece of fruit (apple, orange, banana, peach).

→ Exercise
Gold Standard: 30 minutes of cardio 5 or more days a week
Good Enough: 17 minutes a day
Women who exercised just 2 hours a week (or 17 minutes daily) lowered their risk of stroke and heart disease by 27 percent, according to researchers at Boston's renowned Brigham and Women's Hospital.

→ Staying Hydrated
Gold Standard: eight 8-ounce glasses of water daily
Good Enough: drink with meals and when you're thirsty
If you have trouble getting yourself up to 64 full ounces, take your cue from a National Academy of Sciences panel, which found that women can get adequate fluids (an average of 11 glasses a day) from their usual drinking habits. Simply drink with meals and let your thirst guide you.

→ Strength Training
Gold Standard: two or three times a week
Good Enough: once a week
People who lifted weights just once a week for 2 months gained almost as much lean muscle (3 pounds) as those who hit the weight machines three times per week, one research study found.

→ A Healthy Weight
Gold Standard: BMI between 18 and 25
Good Enough: aim to lose 5 to 7 percent of your current body weight
This degree of weight loss can reduce the risk of diabetes by 58 percent, according to the National Institutes of Health.

My Health Measures Today

It's never too late to start recording your most vital health statistics, especially if you are working to get healthier. Record your initial measurements here to see how you stand up to the healthy levels listed on the previous pages. Then, you can place your ongoing measures in the My Yearly Health Tracker on page 96 or the Daily and Weekly Health Trackers beginning on page 74, depending on your needs and your doctor's instructions. You can also record your health measures online at www.prevention.com/healthtrackers.

DATE:			
Weight		Cholesterol (total)	
BMI		Cholesterol (HDL/LDL)	
Waist circumference		Triglycerides	
Blood pressure		Blood sugar	

BMI

Height	Weight (lbs)													
5'0"	97	102	107	112	118	123	128	133	138	143	148	153	158	163
5'1"	100	106	111	116	122	127	132	137	143	148	153	158	164	169
5'2"	104	109	115	120	126	131	136	142	147	153	158	164	169	175
5'3"	107	113	118	124	130	135	141	146	152	158	163	169	175	180
5'4"	110	116	122	128	134	140	145	151	157	163	169	174	180	186
5'5"	114	120	126	132	138	144	150	156	162	168	174	180	186	192
5'6"	118	124	130	136	142	148	155	161	167	173	179	186	192	198
5'7"	121	127	134	140	146	153	159	166	172	178	185	191	198	204
5'8"	125	131	138	144	151	158	164	171	177	184	190	197	203	210
5'9"	128	135	142	149	155	162	169	176	182	189	196	203	209	216
5'10"	132	139	146	153	160	167	174	181	188	195	202	209	216	222
5'11"	136	143	150	157	165	172	179	186	193	200	208	215	222	229
6'0"	140	147	154	162	169	177	184	191	199	206	213	221	228	235
6'1"	144	151	159	166	174	182	189	197	204	212	219	227	235	242
6'2"	148	155	163	171	179	186	194	202	210	218	225	233	241	249
BMI	19	20	21	22	23	24	25	26	27	28	29	30	31	32

Fitness Tests

WHETHER YOU FOLLOW a prescribed fitness routine, use a trainer, or just love activities that keep your body moving, staying physically active is an essential component of a healthy lifestyle at every age.

Keeping track of your progress over time can keep you motivated by helping you to notice the improvements you've made. Taking these basic measurements will give you a known starting point with which to compare yourself every few weeks as you work toward improving your overall fitness and health. You'll probably want to retest yourself about once a month.

The following tests are intended to measure some fundamentals, including aerobic endurance, strength, and flexibility. You won't need any special gym equipment for the tests below, just a watch with a second hand and a yardstick or tape measure. Don't forget to warm up first—a 5-minute warm-up, including light aerobic activity and some relaxed stretching, will help prevent injuries.

TEST: WALKING

THIS BASIC WALKING TEST is often used to help measure aerobic endurance, or how strong your heart is.

WHAT YOU'LL NEED: a stopwatch (or watch with a second hand) and comfortable walking shoes (preferably sneakers!)

1. Measure a distance of 1 mile. Use the walking maps at www.prevention.com/mywalkingmaps, or go to a local track and determine how many laps constitute 1 mile.

2. Figure out your prewalk heart rate. Sit still for at least 5 minutes in order to get an accurate reading. Press your middle and index fingers on the main artery along the middle of either side of your neck, and count the number of beats you feel for 10 seconds using a stopwatch or second hand. Then multiply by 6 to determine the number of beats per minute.

Heart rate before walk: _______ beats per minute

3. Walk 1 mile as fast as you can. Pace yourself so you can complete the full distance. Of course, if you need to stop and rest along the way, that's okay—just remember that clock needs to keep ticking!

4. Once you've walked the full mile, stop your watch and take note of your complete time. Then immediately take your heart rate a second time.

Time to walk 1 mile: _______ min _______ sec   Heart rate after walk: _______ beats per minute

TEST: STAIR CLIMB

THIS TEST IS A MEASUREMENT of your maximum aerobic capacity, or VO_2 max (volume of oxygen per time measured, which breaks down to milliliters of oxygen used in 1 minute per kilogram of body weight). This measure tells you how efficient your body is at using oxygen at extreme levels of activity. The more oxygen you consume (i.e., the higher your VO_2 max), the more energy you can produce, thus the better your body will perform when physically taxed.

WHAT YOU'LL NEED: a stopwatch (or watch with a second hand) and four flights of stairs (see opposite if you only have one set of stairs)

Climb four flights of stairs (12 to 14 steps each) as fast as you can. If you have only one set, run up and then quickly walk down; repeat for a total of six times. Record your time and heart rate below.

Time to climb four flights: _______ min _______ sec

Heart rate after climbing: _______ beats per minute

TEST: **PUSH-UPS**

THE CLASSIC PUSH-UP is a great way to measure both upper-body strength and muscular endurance, or how long you can do the exercise without getting tired. Get into push-up position, either traditional style with only your hands and toes touching the floor, or in the modified style in which your knees touch the floor to reduce the difficulty of the exercise (either way, be sure to use the same method for follow-up tests!). Your shoulders should be directly over your hands and your body at a 45-degree angle to the floor. Slowly lower your upper body toward the floor, bending your elbows 90 degrees. Straighten your arms and repeat. Do as many push-ups as you can in 1 minute.

Push-ups in 1 minute: _______

TEST: **PLANK**

JUST AS PUSH-UPS MEASURE upper-body endurance, the plank is a good way to determine your core strength endurance. Lie facedown on the floor, and then get into a plank position as follows. Place your forearms on the floor, your elbows under your shoulders, and keep your legs extended behind you. Lift up, balancing on the balls of your feet and your forearms. Keep your abdominals tight to help support your body weight. Hold here for as long as possible, and record your time.

Time in plank position: _______ min _______ sec

TEST: **CHAIR SQUATS**

USE THIS TEST TO HELP evaluate the strength and endurance of your lower-body muscles, especially your quadriceps and glutes. By using a chair, you're able to keep the right form and also determine just how low you need to squat down. Use a standard-size desk chair (no wheels!). Stand a little in front of the chair, feet about hip-distance apart, with arms at sides. Bend your knees, sitting back as if you're about to sit in the chair. Let your butt just lightly touch the seat (don't sit all the way down). Keep your weight over your heels, and don't allow your knees to move past your toes. Stand up and repeat. Do as many squats as you can in 1 minute. If you have to stop and rest, that's okay—but keep that watch running. For best results, use the same chair each time you test yourself.

Squats in 1 minute: _______

TEST: **SIT AND REACH**

THIS IS A CLASSIC TEST to help measure flexibility in the all-too-tight hamstrings and lower back. In order to avoid injuring yourself by stretching cold, be sure to warm up a bit before this test (either by doing the other tests mentioned or by jogging in place).

WHAT YOU'LL NEED: a yardstick or tape measure and some tape

Place the yardstick or tape measure with the zero mark closest to you, and tape it in place at about the 15-inch mark. Sit over the yardstick so it's between your legs, and keep your feet about 12 inches apart, legs straight.

Bring your heels even with the tape at the 15-inch mark. Stack your hands, one over the other, middle fingers aligned and pointing forward. Breathe in, then slowly bend forward as you exhale, being careful not to jerk or bounce your upper body. Slide your fingers along the yardstick as far as possible. Measure how many inches you've moved forward at the farthest point. Repeat a total of three times and record your best result.

Forward reach (best of three tries): _________ inches

TEST: BALANCE DRILLS

ALTHOUGH IT IS SOMETIMES overlooked, balance is often called the "fourth pillar" of fitness, after strength, cardio exercise, and flexibility. It's important in everything we do, especially as we get older. The better your balance, the less likely you are to fall and get injured. Best of all, you'll see improvements in your balance very quickly. Stand tall, feet together and arms at your sides. Lift your right foot a few inches off the floor, either to the side or behind you. Hold here as long as you possibly can. Record your time and repeat with your left leg. Next, do the same exercise with your eyes closed. (You'll be surprised at how much more difficult this becomes!)

Balance time, eyes open (right): _______ min _______ sec; **(left):** _______ min _______ sec

Balance time, eyes closed (right): _______ min _______ sec; **(left):** _______ min _______ sec

The Number on the Scale Isn't Everything!

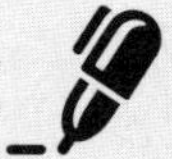

DEPENDING ON your activity level and your body type, your health improvements may not always be apparent if you're only tracking how many pounds you've lost. Because muscle weighs more than fat, your weight may be a misleading indicator of your progress. Also, regular exercise can really reshape your body. Try checking measurements of key points on your body; track them on a chart. Always measure on bare skin to make comparisons easy. For increased accuracy, ask your spouse or a friend to help.

BODY SIZE MEASUREMENTS

Bicep (left): _____________ Bicep (right): _________

Chest: _____________

Waist (just above navel): _____________

Hip (at fullest spot): _____________

Thigh (left): _____________ Thigh (right): _________

Calf (left): _____________ Calf (right): _________

Fitness Test Follow-Ups

Walking Follow-Up

Date	Heart rate (pre)	1 mile walk time	Heart rate (post)

Stair Climb Follow-Up

Date	Stair climb time	Heart rate (post)

Push-Ups Follow-Up

Date	Push-ups per minute

Plank Follow-Up

Date	Time in plank position

Chair Squats Follow-Up

Date	Squats per minute

Sit & Reach Follow-Up

Date	Reach

Balance Drills Follow-Up

Date	Eyes open, R	Eyes open, L	Closed, R	Closed, L

MY HEALTH DECADE BY DECADE

WITH THE RIGHT INFORMATION and support, good health doesn't necessarily have to be a struggle. Follow our decade-by-decade guideposts and stay on the road to vibrant health and long life.

At each life stage, you'll find a Self-Care Checklist, which covers important health issues you might be facing at this point in your life. These include nutritional solutions to problems you may be encountering, as well as tips for improving your physical, mental, and emotional health in a whole variety of ways. You'll also see a First-Time Tests section to explain the purpose of new tests that become important for detecting problems early at each stage and Doctors' Office Checklists outlining which medical tests you should talk with your doctor about scheduling.

Roadblocks to Better Health

WORKING TO IMPROVE your health but running into roadblocks? We have the best tips from top researchers in psychology, weight loss, diet, and exercise to identify the most common goals and the biggest obstacles. Read on to find ways to leap over, duck under, or smash right through those roadblocks!

My Goal: Eat Healthier

- **ROADBLOCK:** "When I get hungry, I always reach for things that taste good but aren't good for me."

  Suzanne Haval Hobbs, DrPH, recommends that you sneak veggies into your fridge in the form of some creamy hummus. Just ½ cup of hummus qualifies as a serving of vegetables! And make a habit of keeping fruit on your desk or kitchen counter.

- **ROADBLOCK:** "I have a sweet tooth."

  If you don't find a way to satisfy it, it'll end up sabotaging your efforts to eat better. Avoid processed foods, which contain artificial sweeteners. Because these sweeteners are processed differently from natural sugar, their effect on your insulin levels may actually prompt you to eat sooner. There are a lot of options for treats that won't have these same effects—check out your local supermarket or natural foods store and seek out more natural alternatives.

My Goal: Get Energized

- **ROADBLOCK:** "I get enough sleep, but I still feel tired."

  There are some straightforward physical problems that could be at the root of this issue. Make a doctor's appointment and get your thyroid and iron levels checked. Try to note when your energy is at its lowest and highest—use your Daily or Weekly Health Trackers—and see if there are any patterns.

• **ROADBLOCK**: "I try to get to sleep at a decent hour, but I still have things that need to be done."

Research has already established the basic methods of improving sleep. Use your bed only for sleep and sex. Remove any televisions or computers. Keep the room cool and dark, and maintain a regular schedule with a consistent time to go to sleep and wake (including weekends!). If you've been in bed for more than 20 minutes without falling asleep, get up and read or do another quiet activity before going back to bed. If you continue to feel stressed or leave tasks undone, consider making use of time management books, consultants, or other resources.

My Goal: **Lose Weight**

• **ROADBLOCK**: "I need more willpower."

Don't worry about willpower—that idea can be more related to guilt or shame than success in achieving one's goals. Instead, set a specific goal and make a plan for reaching it. Instead of telling yourself, "I'll get more exercise this month," decide, "I'll go to step class on Monday nights and go out dancing with my friends on Fridays." With the second goal, you know exactly what you're planning to do and when, and there's more accountability! Give yourself some small rewards for meeting your goals. Then congratulate yourself for any small successes.

• **ROADBLOCK**: "I give up so easily."

Need something tangible to keep you motivated? Check our weight loss simulator at www.prevention.com/mvm/main.html, which will show you what your body will look like when you reach your target weight. And remind yourself that making significant changes in one's life is inherently difficult—you may struggle, and it may take multiple attempts. Cultivate the positive, and focus on the factors that make exercise easier for you—if it works better to go before dinner or to wear your favorite shirt, do that.

My Goal: **Make Exercise a Habit**

• **ROADBLOCK**: "I can't seem to find the time to exercise regularly."

Start small. If your plan is overly ambitious, you might feel overwhelmed before you lace up your sneakers. Plan for a short workout and reward yourself when you succeed. Even 20 minutes of exercise can provide health benefits and help you get a new habit started. A National Institutes of Health study showed that short but frequent workouts (10-minute sessions four times per day) produced the same benefits as one 40-minute workout.

• **ROADBLOCK**: "I want it to be fun."

Anything that gets your heart pumping qualifies as exercise, so consider what activities you already enjoy that involve some physical movement. Enlist a friend or sign up for a class. Once you make a commitment, you'll have some extra incentive to follow through. A University of Florida study found that a better fit between personality and workout led to greater enjoyment of the activity itself. If you're extroverted, you might like high-intensity exercise (try an aerobics class). If you're more anxious or aware of your surroundings, solo activities (treadmill, exercise bike) may be more your style. If you like learning new styles, consider martial arts or dance classes.

MY HEALTH DECADE BY DECADE

THANKS TO IMPROVEMENTS in medicine and technology, as well as a better understanding about what helps us stay healthy, women's life expectancy has increased by nearly 61 percent in the past century, from 48.3 years in 1900 to 79.5 years in 1998. We have more control over the quality of our lives and our health than ever before. An increasing percentage of premature deaths are from preventable causes, including tobacco, poor diet, physical inactivity, alcohol, motor vehicle accidents, drugs, and firearms. Changing habits is much easier at this age than it will be later! Talk to your parents about their family health histories (the charts in My Health History beginning on page 14 will help). Take note of areas that may be potential problems for you, and be sure to inform your doctor(s) so they can advise you.

AGES 18 to 32

Your Self-Care Checklist

☐ **MULTIVITAMINS.** Shore up your dietary needs with a multivitamin and mineral supplement that has:
- 100 percent of the recommended daily value for vitamin A or beta-carotene, vitamin D, vitamin B_6, copper, and zinc
- At least 100 to 500 milligrams of vitamin C and 100 to 400 IU of vitamin E to reduce cell damage and cancer risk

Make sure any vitamins and supplements you take have a USP (United States Pharmacopeia) label, which verifies that the manufacturer guarantees the amount of vitamins listed on the label is accurate.

☐ **BONE HEALTH.** We recommend 500 milligrams of a calcium supplement for all women under 50. Aim for another 500 milligrams per day from calcium-rich foods, such as dark leafy greens and low-fat dairy products.

☐ **IRON LEVELS.** Low iron levels may cause fatigue and trouble concentrating. Boost your iron intake through iron-rich foods like dark green leafy vegetables, legumes, and extra-lean meat—consume with vitamin C–rich foods, like orange juice, to improve your body's ability to absorb the iron. As a backup, consider iron supplements. Speak to your doctor about your iron levels before self-treating.

☐ **GOOD-MOOD FOODS.** A lack of calcium can exacerbate premenstrual symptoms, so be sure you're getting 1,000 milligrams a day via three servings of dairy from milk or yogurt, or from calcium-fortified orange juice.

☐ **OPTIMUM FERTILITY.** One study found that a group of overweight women went from a 75 percent miscarriage rate to an 18 percent rate after exercising, eating a healthy diet, and losing weight. If pregnancy is in your near future, measure your BMI (see page 47) and start working toward a healthy weight.

Also, because folic acid helps to prevent serious birth defects, maximize your intake of the B-vitamin folic acid (we recommend 400 micrograms daily) with two folate-rich foods every day, like orange juice, spinach, or kidney beans. Pregnant women may be advised by their doctors to increase their daily intake to 600 micrograms.

- [ ] **EXERCISE**. It's common to put on a pound a year, and it becomes much more difficult to lose extra weight as you age. Build good exercise habits now to help you maintain a healthy weight and a healthy body throughout your life.

First-Time Tests

- [ ] **BLOOD SUGAR** (fasting blood glucose level): If you're overweight or have other diabetes risk factors, such as high triglycerides, high cholesterol, or a family history, get tested now.

- [ ] **COMPLETE BLOOD LIPID PROFILE:** This test measures cholesterol and triglyceride levels, which are related to illnesses such as heart disease and diabetes. Starting at age 20, get tested at least every 5 years (many physicians run the full profile or a modified version as part of your annual blood work). If your results are abnormal, get tested every 4 months.

- [ ] **ELECTROCARDIOGRAM (EKG):** Get this test done at age 30 to serve as a baseline, so that your doctor can better monitor your heart health later.

- [ ] **STD TESTS**. If you haven't already, as soon as you become sexually active, you should include tests for chlamydia, gonorrhea, and HIV as part of your annual exam.

Your Doctors' Office Checklists

General Practitioner

- [ ] **SERUM FERRITIN TEST AND TRANSFERRIN SATURATION TEST:** Screening suggested at age 18 to check for iron deficiency

- [ ] **EKG:** At age 30 for a baseline

- [ ] **BLOOD PRESSURE CHECK:** Every 2 years

- [ ] **FASTING GLUCOSE TEST:** Now if you're at high risk, and every 3 years

- [ ] **SKIN EXAM:** Every 3 years, every year if skin cancer runs in your family, or twice a year if you're at high risk

- [ ] **COMPLETE BLOOD LIPID PROFILE:** Every 5 years, starting at age 20; if results are abnormal, go every 4 months

- [ ] **TETANUS SHOT:** Every 10 years

- [ ] **HEARING TEST:** Every 10 years

Obstetrician/Gynecologist

- [ ] **PELVIC EXAM AND PAP TEST:** Every year

- [ ] **CLINICAL BREAST EXAM:** Every year

- [ ] **STD TESTS**. As soon as you become sexually active, and annually thereafter

Dentist

- [ ] **DENTAL CHECKUPS:** Every 6 months

Optometrist

- [ ] **EYE EXAMS:** Get an initial comprehensive exam and follow up if you notice vision changes.

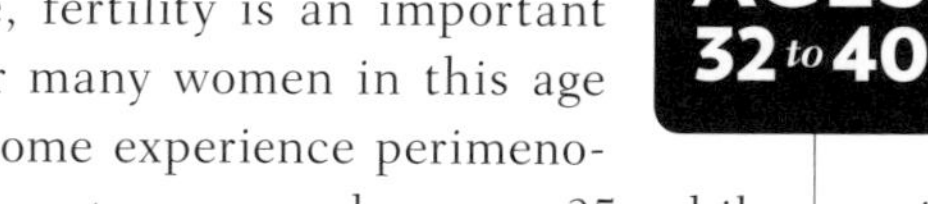

EVEN IF YOU'VE ALREADY established a healthy lifestyle, now is the time to deal with specific changes that typically occur as women approach midlife. For instance, fertility is an important issue for many women in this age group. Some experience perimenopausal symptoms as early as age 35, while others won't see them until their late forties. Also, beginning in their thirties, women lose 1 to 2 percent of their muscle mass per year, but exercise can reverse the process and keep your metabolism up. Weight-bearing exercise, such as walking and lifting weights, will strengthen your skeleton and help you avoid osteoporosis, heart disease, diabetes, and a host of other health problems.

Your Self-Care Checklist

☐ **MULTIVITAMINS.** Just as you did in your twenties, shore up your dietary needs with a multivitamin and mineral supplement that has:
  • 100 percent of the recommended daily value for vitamin A or beta-carotene, vitamin D, vitamin B_6, copper, and zinc
  • At least 100 to 500 milligrams of vitamin C and 100 to 400 IU of vitamin E to reduce cell damage and cancer risk
  Make sure any vitamins and supplements you take have a USP (United States Pharmacopeia) label, which verifies that the manufacturer guarantees the amount of vitamins listed on the label is accurate.

☐ **FOLATE FOR CELLULAR HEALTH.** Folate works to keep your DNA strong and also decreases your risk of colon cancer. Increase your intake with foods such as spinach, legumes, and other vegetables and fruits. The suggested daily value (DV) for women is 400 micrograms of folic acid (the supplement form of folate).

☐ **BONE HEALTH.** These recommendations are the same as they were for your twenties. We recommend 500 milligrams of a calcium supplement for all women under 50. Aim for another 500 milligrams per day from calcium-rich foods, such as dark leafy greens and low-fat dairy products, and get plenty of exercise to help keep your bones strong.

☐ **OPTIMUM FERTILITY.** Just as in your twenties, measuring your BMI (see page 47) and working toward a healthy weight may increase your chances of pregnancy.
  Also, maximize your intake of the B-vitamin folic acid (we recommend 400 micrograms daily) with two folate-rich foods every day, like orange juice, spinach, or kidney beans. Pregnant women may be advised by their doctors to increase their daily intake to 600 micrograms.

☐ **EXERCISE.** If you aren't already exercising on a regular basis, start now. Proper exercise also improves flexibility and heart and other muscle strength and is a key factor in maintaining a healthy weight (your metabolism begins to slow in your thirties, making it easier to gain weight).

First-Time Tests

- [ ] **TSH SCREENING.** The American Thyroid Association recommends checking your thyroid-stimulating hormone levels at age 35 and at least every 5 years thereafter. Schedule an additional test if you have gained or lost weight rapidly or if your energy level has been very low.

- [ ] **BONE DENSITY TEST.** If you're at high risk for osteoporosis, your doctor might recommend that you get a screening now instead of in your late forties. Be sure you're aware of your family history and any other risk factors, and talk to your doctor.

- [ ] **MAMMOGRAM.** If you're at high risk for breast cancer, your doctor might recommend that you get a screening now instead of in your forties. Be sure you're aware of your family history and any other risk factors, and talk to your doctor.

Your Doctors' Office Checklists

General Practitioner

- [ ] **SERUM FERRITIN TEST AND TRANSFERRIN SATURATION TEST:** Ask your physician about current recommendations for these tests to check for iron deficiency.

- [ ] **BLOOD PRESSURE CHECK:** Every 2 years, or more frequently if it's been abnormal

- [ ] **FASTING GLUCOSE TEST:** Every 3 years, more frequently if you're at high risk. (Women in their thirties and early forties who have battled weight problems are at high risk for prediabetes, a dangerous condition that indicates they're very close to developing diabetes. If you're overweight or have other risk factors, such as high triglycerides, high cholesterol, or a family history, get tested.)

- [ ] **SKIN EXAM:** Every 3 years, every year if skin cancer runs in your family, or twice a year if you're at high risk

- [ ] **COMPLETE BLOOD LIPID PROFILE:** Every 2 years starting at age 35, with abnormal results rechecked every 4 months

- [ ] **TETANUS SHOT:** If it's been 10 years, get another one.

- [ ] **HEARING TEST:** If it's been 10 years, get another one.

- [ ] **THYROID-STIMULATING HORMONE TEST:** Every 5 years

- [ ] **BONE DENSITY TEST:** If you're at high risk for osteoporosis, get a baseline bone density scan prior to menopause. Otherwise, wait until menopause for the test.

Obstetrician/Gynecologist

- [ ] **PELVIC EXAM AND PAP TEST:** Every year

- [ ] **CLINICAL BREAST EXAM:** Every year, and do monthly breast self-exams

- [ ] **STD TESTS:** Every year

- [ ] **MAMMOGRAM:** If two or more close relatives had breast cancer, particularly before they turned 40, start annual mammograms in your thirties. Otherwise, it can wait until your forties.

Dentist

- [ ] **DENTAL CHECKUPS:** Every 6 months

Optometrist

- [ ] **EYE EXAMS:** Schedule a comprehensive eye exam, especially if you've never had one or if you notice a change in your vision.

MY HEALTH DECADE BY DECADE

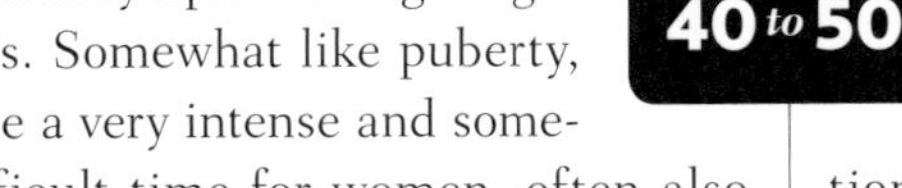

AT THIS STAGE OF LIFE, many women experience some health-related challenges, particularly as menopause approaches. Eighty-five to 90 percent of women experience symptoms of perimenopause, the most common symptom being irregular periods. Somewhat like puberty, this can be a very intense and sometimes difficult time for women, often also characterized by significant life changes. Continuing to build your healthy body with good food and essential supplements, along with scheduling all necessary medical tests, will help you get to any potential problems as early as possible. And, if you begin finding it easier to put weight on and harder to take it off, you're not alone! Metabolism slows down as you age, and lower rates of estrogen production may also affect your weight. If you haven't built up a habit of regular exercise, start now—it's never too late.

Your Self-Care Checklist

☐ **MULTIVITAMINS.** Take a multivitamin and mineral supplement to ensure that you get 100 percent of the recommended daily value for the most important nutrients. Talk with your doctor about what amounts of particular vitamins and minerals are recommended for your age group (some suggestions are listed here) or to help with your individual health concerns. Make sure any vitamins and supplements you take have a USP (United States Pharmacopeia) label, which verifies that the manufacturer guarantees the amount of vitamins listed on the label is accurate.

☐ **PERIMENOPAUSE SYMPTOMS.** Cool hot flashes, relieve mood swings, and soothe vaginal dryness with 800 IU of a vitamin E daily supplement. To further reduce perimenopause symptoms, eat whole grain bread and cereals, as well as fruits and vegetables. In addition to their other nutrients, these foods provide fiber, which helps balance your estrogen levels.

☐ **BONE HEALTH.** As you've read in other sections, we recommend 500 milligrams of a calcium supplement for all women under 50. Taken with a diet that includes low-fat dairy (such as cheese and yogurt) and dark leafy-green vegetables, you'll have all the calcium you need for keeping bones strong without the saturated fat.

☐ **NATURAL FOODS.** Processed foods tend to be full of empty calories, lacking in vitamins, minerals, and fiber but packing a lot of fat and sugar. Because you need fewer calories as you age, get the most out of the ones you do eat by choosing natural foods, which are higher in nutrients.

☐ **CALORIE CONTROL.** Experiment with small changes, like eliminating just a bite of every meal. That alone will add up to 100 fewer calories each day.

☐ **HUNGER SIGNALS.** As your body's needs change, it's important to pay attention to your hunger signals and your body's response to food. Eat slowly, being mindful of how food makes you feel. Note how you feel the rest of the day, and pay special attention to recurring patterns. Keeping track of your food intake in a log can be particularly helpful (check out the Daily and Weekly Health Trackers on pages 74 through 91).

☐ **EXERCISE, EXERCISE, EXERCISE.** Women tend to gain about a pound a year in their forties, so be sure to keep your exercise program going. Weight gain at this age can be a particular problem because women become more likely to add fat to the abdomen, where it will do more damage to blood sugar, blood pressure, and cholesterol levels.

☐ **FLU SHOTS.** Whether you're in good health or your health is compromised, get a flu shot in September or October every year to help avoid coming down with the most prevalent strains of the flu virus. (If you're allergic to eggs, check with your doctor first!)

First-Time Tests

☐ **STRESS ECHOCARDIOGRAM AND EKG:** Researchers have found that heart disease is increasingly diagnosed at younger ages in women. Incorporate a stress echocardiogram and EKG into your regular test regimen, particularly if you're at high risk of heart disease due to lifestyle, family history, or ethnicity (a 20-year University of California, San Francisco, study of more than 5,000 people found that young African-Americans were 20 times as likely as young Caucasians to experience heart failure).

☐ **MAMMOGRAM.** Although breast cancer is still rare for women in their forties (less than 2 percent are affected), the importance of catching problems early means that you should start screening annually if you haven't already because of high risk factors.

☐ **BONE DENSITY TEST.** If you haven't already had one, schedule this test as soon as you begin to see signs of menopause. If you're at risk for osteoporosis (see "Beyond Calcium" on page 60), get tested right away.

☐ **PELVIC ULTRASOUND.** A pelvic ultrasound will catch ovarian cancer early. Schedule one now if you have a family history or other risk factors.

"Health is not valued till sickness comes."

—DR. THOMAS FULLER

Beyond Calcium: Maintain Bone Health in Your Forties

KEEP AN EYE ON your menstrual cycle. Missed periods are a sign of perimenopause, during which it's critical to increase efforts to keep your bones healthy.

→ **Incorporate strength training into your exercise regimen.** Strength training is vital for maintaining bone and muscle strength. Other kinds of weight-bearing exercise, including walking, are also healthy. Check out www.prevention.com/health/fitness/walking for tips on how to create fun, invigorating walking workouts.

→ **Evaluate your risk.** Let your doctor know about your risk factors (smoking, a family history of osteoporosis or fractures, suffering a fracture yourself as an adult, going through menopause before age 40, having had an eating disorder, or being underweight), and consider having an early bone density test.

→ **Pay attention to back pain.** Sudden back pain may be caused by a vertebral fracture, which becomes more common as women approach the age of 50 but often goes undiagnosed.

→ **Monitor your overall health.** Other health problems, including an overactive thyroid or the onset of type 2 diabetes, can affect your bones. These problems become more common in your forties, so stay up to date on recommended tests.

Your Doctors' Office Checklists

General Practitioner

- ☐ **SERUM FERRITIN TEST AND TRANSFERRIN SATURATION TEST:** Ask your physician about current recommendations for these tests to check for iron deficiency.

- ☐ **BLOOD PRESSURE CHECK:** Every 2 years, or more frequently if it's been abnormal

- ☐ **FASTING GLUCOSE TEST:** Every 3 years

- ☐ **SKIN EXAM:** Annually

- ☐ **COMPLETE BLOOD LIPID PROFILE:** Every 2 years, with abnormal results rechecked every 4 months

- ☐ **TETANUS SHOT:** If it's been 10 years, get another one.

- ☐ **HEARING TEST:** If it's been 10 years, get another one.

- ☐ **THYROID-STIMULATING HORMONE TEST:** Every 5 years

- ☐ **FLU SHOT:** Every year in September or October

- ☐ **BONE DENSITY TEST:** If you're at high risk for osteoporosis or at the first signs of menopause, get a bone density scan.

- ☐ **STRESS ECHOCARDIOGRAM AND EKG:** At least once and as recommended by your doctor.

Obstetrician/Gynecologist

- ☐ **PELVIC EXAM AND PAP TEST:** Every year

- ☐ **CLINICAL BREAST EXAM:** Every year, and do monthly breast self-exams.

- ☐ **STD TESTS:** If you've been with the same sexual partner and had normal Pap tests for the last 3 years, get tested every 2 to 3 years. Otherwise continue testing every year.

- ☐ **MAMMOGRAM:** Every year

- ☐ **PELVIC ULTRASOUND:** If you're at high risk for ovarian cancer, have a pelvic ultrasound and a CA-125 test, which looks for cancer markers in the blood.

Dentist

- ☐ **DENTAL CHECKUPS:** Every 6 months

Optometrist

- ☐ **EYE EXAMS:** Every 2 to 4 years, or sooner if you notice a change in your vision.

Meditation for Busy Women

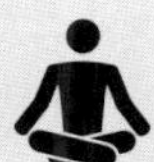 YOU'RE PROBABLY AWARE of the many benefits of meditation, including stress reduction, better concentration, and an improved immune system, among others. There are many centuries of teaching about correct postures and techniques, but you can begin to reap the benefits of meditation with just a few simple tips.

→ **Lower your expectations of meditation.** Commit to 10 minutes a day in which you'll sit still and remain present, focusing on your breathing. Simply observe what happens in your mind and body during this time.

→ **Try to focus on your breathing.** If you happen to notice your mind wandering off, just imagine touching the thoughts lightly or blowing them away, and bring your focus back to your breath. You don't have to start over.

→ **Watch for something surprising.** Our brain whirlwind often distracts us from thoughts or feelings that make us uncomfortable, like worries or minor pains, which can be helpful in the short-term. But eventually we need to know what these anxiety-provoking feelings are so we can resolve them. When your mind is quiet, these issues often reassert themselves. Be open to nontraditional methods of meditation. The essence of meditation is mindful awareness of the present. This can be done during many activities, including exercising, showering, eating, playing or listening to music, drawing, and knitting, among others.

my current health

MANY WOMEN FIND themselves feeling better and more in control in their fifties than they ever have before. At this point you've come to understand what makes you feel happy and fulfilled, and you're more willing to push for it. You can also look forward to relief from perimenopausal symptoms. After 12 months without a period, you've officially reached menopause, which could happen anywhere between the ages of 40 and 58 (average age: 51). But with the relief also comes new health challenges. Women can lose between 2 to 5 percent of bone mass on average per year in the first 3 to 5 years after menopause. While estrogen protected you from heart disease in younger years, losing it in menopause raises LDL ("bad") cholesterol levels. Estrogen also kept your blood vessels naturally elastic. Without it, the risk of both heart disease and stroke increases. Heart disease is one of the primary killers of women, and the majority of women who develop it will begin to experience symptoms during their fifties. For these reasons, a healthy diet, daily exercise, and regular screenings are especially important at this age. These habits will also protect against cancer, arthritis, and other diseases.

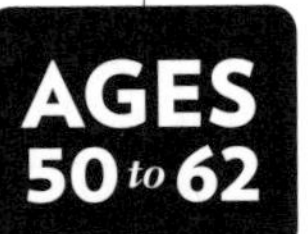

Your Self-Care Checklist

☐ **MULTIVITAMINS.** As in earlier decades, take a multivitamin and mineral supplement to ensure that you get 100 percent of the recommended daily value for the most important nutrients. However, many manufacturers make multivitamins specifically for the 50+ crowd. Ask your doctor what amounts of which vitamins and minerals are recommended for your age group (some suggestions are listed here) or to help with your individual health concerns. Make sure any vitamins and supplements you take have a USP (United States Pharmacopeia) label, which verifies that the manufacturer guarantees the amount of vitamins listed on the label is accurate.

☐ **HEART HEALTH.** Take your B_{12} in a multivitamin supplement—just 6 micrograms per day will help your body fight heart disease.

☐ **EYE STRENGTH.** To protect your retina from age-related macular degeneration, eat spinach daily—it contains the antioxidants lutein and zeaxanthin. Because fat promotes lutein absorption, eat your spinach with olive oil.

☐ **LOW-FAT, HIGH-FIBER DIET.** Reduce your risk of colon and breast cancers, heart disease, and a range of other health problems by stocking up on whole grain breads and cereals, legumes, fruits, vegetables, and fat-free dairy foods.

☐ **CALORIE REDUCTION.** As your metabolism continues to slow, cut your daily calorie intake by at least 100 calories.

☐ **MINI-MEALS.** Eat six smaller meals of about 250 calories each (instead of three big ones) to keep your metabolism going strong.

☐ **BONE HEALTH.** Increase your daily consumption of calcium to 1,200 milligrams, 700 milligrams of which can be in supplement form.

☐ **FALL PREVENTION**. Evaluate the safety of your home and other locations you often visit. Consider adding a stronger handrail or making other changes in order to keep safe.

☐ **FLU SHOT**. Everyone over age 50 should get a flu shot each September or October to reduce the risk of what can be a deadly disease at this age. (If you're allergic to eggs, check with your doctor first!)

First-Time Tests

☐ **COLORECTAL CANCER SCREENING**. There are several tests for colorectal cancer, including a fecal occult blood test (FOBT), digital rectal exam, sigmoidoscopy, colonoscopy, and double contrast barium enema (DCBE). Schedule your first screening by age 50, or earlier if you have a family history or other risk factors (such as gastrointestinal problems). Your doctor will help determine which test is right for you.

☐ **VITAMIN D SCREENING**. Vitamin D deficiency is a major issue in patients with persistent musculoskeletal pain and other joint and bone disorders. Get screened by age 50, and take vitamin D supplements to maintain a healthy level.

Expand Your Horizons

AS WE AGE, we often withdraw from others, spending time with a shrinking circle of friends and family. To counteract the increasing isolation that comes with advancing age in the United States, make an effort to find new sources of joy in your life. Check out social networking Web sites like www.meetup.com, which are designed to connect people with similar interests and facilitate in-person meetings. Or simply peruse the bulletin board at your local library or supermarket and look for classes or activities that catch your eye. Make it a goal to find one new activity this year, even if it takes a few tries to find the right place for you.

Your Doctors' Office Checklists

General Practitioner

- ☐ **SERUM FERRITIN TEST AND TRANSFERRIN SATURATION TEST**: Ask your physician about current recommendations for these tests to check for iron deficiency.

- ☐ **BLOOD PRESSURE CHECK**: Every 2 years, or more frequently if it's been abnormal

- ☐ **FASTING GLUCOSE TEST**: Every 3 years

- ☐ **SKIN EXAM**: Annually

- ☐ **COMPLETE BLOOD LIPID PROFILE**: Every 2 years, with abnormal results rechecked every 4 months

- ☐ **TETANUS SHOT**: If it's been 10 years, get another one.

- ☐ **HEARING TEST**: Every 3 years

- ☐ **THYROID-STIMULATING HORMONE TEST**: Every 5 years

- ☐ **FLU SHOT**: Every year in September or October

Women, Heart Disease, and Stroke

HEART DISEASE is the number one killer of women and stroke is number three on the list. Because the risk factors for heart disease and preventable stroke types are almost identical, you can greatly improve your chances of avoiding these two major health issues at once.

While women and men share the same risk factors (high cholesterol, high blood pressure, diabetes, smoking, overweight and obesity, poor diet, physical inactivity, alcohol use, and high stress), women have an important additional risk factor: menopause. Estrogen, which protects you from heart disease by keeping down cholesterol in your body (especially LDL, "bad" cholesterol) and maintaining blood vessel elasticity, decreases in menopause. Menopausal women are twice as likely to develop heart disease as women of the same age who are not yet menopausal.

Women are also more likely to die from heart disease at this age than men. According to the National Heart, Lung, and Blood Institute, two-thirds of all women who have a heart attack fail to make a full recovery. Nearly a quarter will die within 1 year.

One problem has been that women experience symptoms of heart disease differently than men. Instead of traditional red flags such as chest pain, cold sweats, and numbness or pain in the left arm, women tend to experience breathlessness; nausea or vomiting; clamminess; fatigue and weakness; pressure in the lower chest that can be mistaken for indigestion; and pain in the upper back, shoulders, neck, or jaw. It's common for women and their doctors to dismiss these symptoms as unimportant. (Stroke symptoms are the same in women as they are in men. See pages 30 to 31 for more information on important symptoms.)

Having just one risk factor doubles your likelihood of developing heart disease, so while you can't control your family history, watching your lipoprotein profile, fasting glucose, blood pressure, and BMI along with regular doctor visits (and quitting smoking!) will help you control your risk for heart disease and stroke. It's never too late to choose a healthy life!

- ☐ **BONE DENSITY TEST**: Get a bone density measurement if you're in menopause or past menopause and you've never had a test.

- ☐ **STRESS ECHOCARDIOGRAM AND EKG**: At least once and as recommended by your doctor

- ☐ **HEIGHT MEASUREMENT**: Get measured at each doctor's visit, or at least once a year.

- ☐ **25-HYDROXY VITAMIN D SERUM LEVEL CHECK**: If you're older than 49, have your vitamin D level checked.

- ☐ **COLORECTAL CANCER SCREENING**: Ask for a digital rectal exam and a colonoscopy at age 50 and every 10 years thereafter—or ask your doctor if you can opt for flexible sigmoidoscopy every 3 to 5 years. Also get a yearly fecal occult blood test.

- ☐ **LOW-DOSE CAT SCAN**: If you're 60 or older and smoke now or have smoked in the past, get screened for lung cancer.

Obstetrician/Gynecologist

- ☐ **PELVIC EXAM AND PAP TEST**: Every year

- ☐ **CLINICAL BREAST EXAM**: Every year, and do monthly breast self-exams

- ☐ **STD TESTS**: If you have been with the same sexual partner and had normal Pap tests for the last 3 years, you can take these safely every 2 to 3 years. Otherwise, continue to get tested every year.

- ☐ **MAMMOGRAM**: Every year

- ☐ **PELVIC ULTRASOUND**: If you're at high risk for ovarian cancer, have a pelvic ultrasound and a CA-125 test, a blood test that looks for cancer markers in the blood.

Dentist

- ☐ **DENTAL CHECKUPS**: Every 6 months

Optometrist

- ☐ **EYE EXAMS**: Every 2 to 4 years or sooner if you notice a change in your vision

"There is a healthy way to be ill."

—GEORGE SHEEHAN, MD

MY HEALTH DECADE BY DECADE

WOMEN IN THEIR SIXTIES face unique health concerns, including the increased importance of screenings to catch any potential problems before they become serious. Mammograms and screens for colon cancer are now absolutely necessary, and it's important to continue your regular gynecological visits as well. Exercise should continue to be a high priority, keeping your bones and muscles strong, burning extra calories, and helping to improve your mood. Plus, exercise will continue to help you keep your weight under control, which in turn helps you avoid pain in your hips, knees, ankles, and feet. Staying active in general will keep you emotionally connected to others; the need to connect emotionally with friends and family is just as important as the need to keep your body healthy with good food and exercise and your mind healthy with new challenges and experiences.

AGES 62+

Your Self-Care Checklist

☐ **MULTIVITAMINS.** As with earlier decades, continue taking a multivitamin and mineral supplement to ensure that you get 100 percent of the recommended daily value for the most important nutrients. Many manufacturers make multivitamins specifically for the 50+ crowd. Ask your doctor what amounts of which vitamins and minerals are recommended for your age group (some suggestions are listed here) or to help with your individual health concerns. Make sure any vitamins and supplements you take have a USP (United States Pharmacopeia) label, which verifies that the manufacturer guarantees the amount of vitamins listed on the label is accurate.

☐ **HEART HEALTH.** Take your B_{12} in a mulitvitamin supplement—just 6 micrograms per day will help your body fight heart disease. This recommendation is the same as it was for your fifties.

☐ **ANTIOXIDANT-RICH FOOD.** Stimulate your immune system and fend off cellular degeneration with the antioxidants found in fruits, vegetables, and whole grains.

☐ **NUTRIENT-DENSE FOOD.** Whole grains, beans, low-fat dairy, fruits and vegetables, and small amounts of extra-lean meat will help you make every calorie count!

☐ **RESTAURANT CHOICES.** Look for "light" entrées, fat-free condiment options, and whenever possible order low-fat choices such as plain burgers or grilled chicken at fast-food restaurants. To cut portions, request that half the meal be wrapped to go before it's set down in front of you.

☐ **BONE HEALTH.** As in your fifties, maintain your daily consumption of calcium at 1,200 milligrams, 700 milligrams of which can be in supplement form.

☐ **FALL PREVENTION.** This recommendation is the same as for your fifties. As you age, your bones become more brittle, making you prone to bone breaks and injury, which can influence or cause many different health problems. Continue to ensure that your home and other locations you often visit are safe and offer supports such as handrails and smooth, ramped passages.

☐ **FLU SHOT.** Everyone over age 50—except those allergic to eggs or the flu vaccine—should get a flu shot each September or October to reduce the risk of infection with what can be a deadly disease at this age.

☐ **PNEUMOCOCCAL VACCINE.** The Centers for Disease Control and Prevention (CDC) recommends this vaccine for all adults over the age of 65, as they are more likely to suffer complications if they become ill. Speak to your doctor about getting the vaccine this year.

~~~~~~

Fall Prevention 101

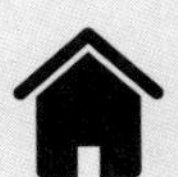

THROUGHOUT YOUR HOME, make sure carpets and rugs are firmly tacked down and noncarpeted areas have no-slip strips. Consider rearranging furniture to create unobstructed walking paths. Run cords and wires along the walls. Keep emergency numbers in large print near each telephone, and don't take risks—it's better to ask for help than to fall and break a bone. Some room-specific tips:

→ **Bedroom:** Put night lights, light switches, and your phone close to your bed.

→ **Bathroom:** Install support bars near your toilet and both inside and outside your tub/shower. In the tub/shower, use a bathing chair or stool and buy soap on a rope.

→ **Stairs and hallways:** Install handrails on both sides. All passages should be well lit with light switches at the top and bottom of stairs and at each end of a long hall.

→ **Kitchen:** Keep things you use regularly in low cabinets or on tabletops. If you need something stored higher, use a special "reach stick" or a step-stool with a handrail.
~~~~~~

First-Time Tests

☐ **EYE EXAMS.** Even if your vision is still normal, it's important to be screened for cataracts, glaucoma, and macular degeneration at this age.

Your Doctors' Office Checklists

General Practitioner

☐ **SERUM FERRITIN TEST AND TRANSFERRIN SATURATION TEST:** Ask your physician about current recommendations for these tests to check for iron deficiency.

☐ **BLOOD PRESSURE CHECK:** Every 2 years, or more frequently if it's been abnormal

☐ **FASTING GLUCOSE TEST:** Every 3 years

☐ **SKIN EXAM:** Annually

☐ **COMPLETE BLOOD LIPID PROFILE:** Every 2 years, with abnormal results rechecked every 4 months

☐ **TETANUS SHOT:** If it's been 10 years, get another one.

☐ **HEARING TEST:** Every 3 years or sooner if you notice changes to your hearing

☐ **THYROID-STIMULATING HORMONE TEST:** Every 5 years

Maintaining Physical and Emotional Vitality

WE PAY A LOT OF ATTENTION to our bodies—all those tests, screenings, quizzes, and questions add up to a whole lot of effort. But sometimes we forget how closely tied our emotional, mental, and physical lives really are. Have you ever noticed that when you're in a bad mood, that banged thumb seems to hurt a lot more than usual (or that you're more prone to banging it)? Or how much more tired you feel when you haven't been able to spend time with a friend or loved one? Our mental and emotional states are as much a part of our health as our physical body, so be sure to take care of all of them as you age!

➔ **Replace "lost" activities.** If you're no longer able to run, try walking or swimming. If you've enjoyed social activities like dancing, consider another activity, like an aerobics class. Replacing activities you've enjoyed can help reduce the loss of control that some people feel as they age.

➔ **Stay physically active.** Incorporate walking into your daily routine, and explore other activities that keep your energy level up and help combat emotional struggles like anxiety and depression, as well as reduce your risk of dementia and Alzheimer's disease.

➔ **Stay sharp.** Maintain or improve your mental dexterity by challenging your intellect on a daily basis. Try learning a new skill, like playing an instrument. Puzzles and strategy games can keep your brain active, which will keep you building brain power instead of losing it.

➔ **Be social.** Stay in touch with friends and family, and continue building connections in your community. Consider volunteering even a small amount of time each week or month. If you feel connected to others, you're more likely to remain healthy.

- ☐ **FLU SHOT**: Every year in September or October

- ☐ **BONE DENSITY TEST**: Be screened regularly and tested every 3 to 5 years.

- ☐ **STRESS ECHOCARDIOGRAM AND EKG**: At least once and as recommended by your doctor

- ☐ **HEIGHT MEASUREMENT**: Get measured at each doctor's visit, or at least once a year.

- ☐ **25-HYDROXY VITAMIN D SERUM LEVEL CHECK**: If you're older than 49, have your vitamin D level checked.

- ☐ **COLORECTAL SCREENING**: Get a digital rectal exam every year and a colonoscopy every 10 years, along with a yearly fecal occult blood test. If you don't have risk factors for colon cancer, you can request a flexible sigmoidoscopy every 3 to 5 years instead of a colonoscopy.

- ☐ **LOW-DOSE CAT SCAN**: If you're 60 or older and smoke now or have smoked in the past, get screened for lung cancer.

Obstetrician/Gynecologist

- ☐ **PELVIC EXAM AND PAP TEST**: Every year

- ☐ **CLINICAL BREAST EXAM**: Every year, and do monthly breast self-exams

- ☐ **STD TESTS**: If you have been with the same sexual partner and had normal Pap tests for the last 3 years, you can take these safely every 2 to 3 years. Otherwise, continue to get tested every year.

- ☐ **MAMMOGRAM**: Every year

- ☐ **PELVIC ULTRASOUND**: If you're at high risk for ovarian cancer, have a pelvic ultrasound and a CA-125 test, a blood test that looks for cancer markers in the blood.

Dentist

- ☐ **DENTAL CHECKUPS**: Every 6 months

Optometrist

- ☐ **EYE EXAMS**: After you turn 65, start going to the eye doctor every year, or go sooner if you notice a change in your vision.

> **"It's no longer a question of staying healthy. It's a question of finding a sickness you like."**
>
> —JACKIE MASON, COMEDIAN

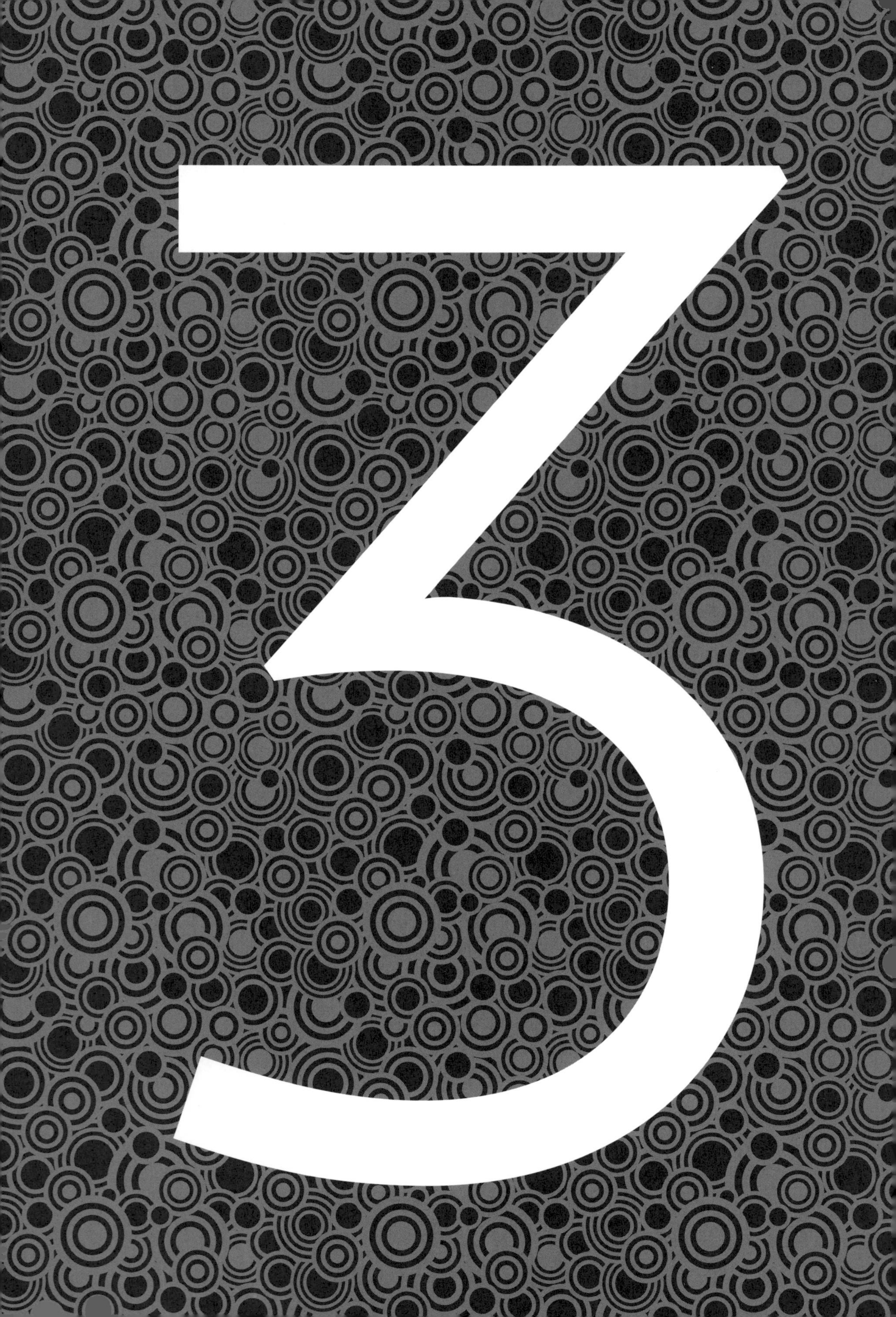

MY HEALTH JOURNAL

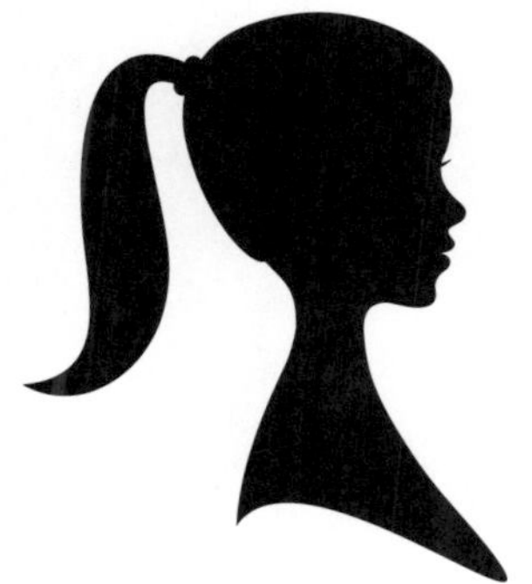

KEEPING A JOURNAL has been shown to have a powerful impact on everything from reaching weight loss goals to relieving depression. The act of writing things down raises your awareness of the millions of biological interactions that happen in your body and mind. In this section, we give you space to record what you do—and the effect it has on your health. We've given you a few different options because some people prefer to journal every day while others find that to be too often. Also, you may want to record some measurements every day but others only once a year. Use as many as you find helpful, and feel free to photocopy the trackers you find most helpful.

> **"Learning is not attained by chance, it must be sought for with ardor and attended to with diligence."**
> —ABIGAIL ADAMS

MY HEALTH TRACKERS

T'S OFTEN BEEN OBSERVED that information isn't considered important—and can't be used—until it's measured. That's why we've developed this section to provide a place for you to measure and then track your way to healthier habits from now into the long term. With these charts, you can keep all of your important health information together in one place to easily monitor changes and take note of important health events over time.

It turns out that one of the most powerful tools available for losing weight and generally improving health may be your pen and paper. A Kaiser Permanente study involving more than 1,600 people found that over a 6-month period, those who kept a food journal lost twice as much weight as those who did not.

Why is this so effective? Experts agree that both increased personal accountability and a greater awareness of patterns, habits, and traps are the primary factors. Our memories are notoriously inaccurate, and those unreliable accounts of the past make it harder for us to realize that changes may be necessary. Records like these make patterns easier to see and help you notice more quickly when a problem is developing. Noticing how negative effects often follow certain behaviors, such as observing that you tend to gain weight when you're depressed or that a lack of sleep makes you feel more irritable, can help you break destructive patterns and exchange unhealthy habits for healthier ones. When you have all the information in front of you, it's easier to understand how you might adapt in order to meet your goals.

Here's a tip: For the first week or two, simply keep a record of your current behavior. You may find that the increased attention prompts change even at this early stage. Then, after you have

Weighing Daily: Help or Hindrance?

BROWN UNIVERSITY researchers found that dieters were more likely to keep weight off if they weighed themselves daily, but only if they used the information to make changes, like incrementally adjusting their exercise level or making better food choices. Consider recording your weight each time you weigh yourself to make it easier to observe long-term trends. The technique can backfire, however, if frequent weigh-ins cause you to become discouraged or to obsess about your weight. If you've had an eating disorder, definitely stay away from those daily trips to the scale. And remember, your weight fluctuates naturally. Don't become concerned until the weight gain approaches 5 pounds. However often you weigh yourself, make sure it's always under the same circumstances; for example, always early in the morning, after you've gone to the bathroom but before eating or exercising. Be sure to note changes around your period, but don't be too concerned about an extra pound or two during that time—these are likely temporary.

Three Good Things

RESEARCHERS FOUND that people who wrote down three things that went well each day, along with a causal explanation for each thing, showed significantly greater levels of happiness up to 6 months after the exercise ended! Make yourself more aware of the good things that happen each day, and train your brain to pay attention to the positive by adopting this simple daily practice. Each day before you go to bed, write down three good things that happened (try using your Daily or Weekly Health Tracker). Be as specific as possible. Instead of writing general statements like "I have great friends," pin down exactly what happened that day to remind you of these things. For example, "I enjoyed seeing my friend at lunch today, and I noticed how much better I felt after spending time with her." For each positive event you write down, answer the question, "Why did this good thing happen?" Over time, you might begin to see patterns that will help you understand what people, experiences, or environments tend to lead to positive experiences for you.

---

your baseline, set a goal that will be relatively easy to reach, and choose a small reward that will help motivate you. When you're trying to establish a new pattern, rewards can be a big help. Begin with your most important goal, whether it's getting more sleep, losing weight, flattening your belly, or eating more fruits and vegetables. Continue monitoring yourself, and consider including additional variables that may be related to your goal. If you understand how other aspects of your life are related to your target behavior, you'll be better prepared to spot problems and make adjustments.

The most important thing is just to get started! For some measurements, such as what you've eaten and how much you've exercised, you'll want to track the details every day; just photocopy the Daily Health Tracker on page 75 as many times as you need (we've provided 1 week's worth of pages). If taking notes every day proves to be too much for you, try the Weekly Health Tracker on page 84; again, photocopy as many times as you need (we've provided 1 month's worth of pages). For longer-term measurements, such as your blood pressure and cholesterol levels—and to see the long-term effects of your daily health habits—use the Yearly Health Tracker on page 96; we've provided 5 years' worth of pages. For each of these tracker pages, we've filled in a sample to give you an idea of how detailed you may want to be.

And if you need more space or just prefer a virtual environment, visit our online tools at www.prevention.com/healthtrackers. Also, don't forget the Fitness Tests beginning on page 48—each includes space to track follow-up tests, but you can always track your results here as well.

 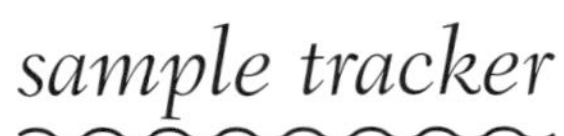

MY DAILY HEALTH TRACKER

GOAL: *2 servings fruit, 3 servings vegetables*   **REWARD:** *long, hot bath*

DATE: *1/5/11*   **WEIGHT:** *156 lbs*   **HOURS OF SLEEP:** *7*

Foods Eaten

Time	Food	Amount/Unit	Carbs	Fat	Protein	Calories
Breakfast 7:30 a.m.	Orange juice	1 cup	26 g	0	2 g	112
	Whole wheat toast	2 slices	26 g	2 g	8 g	152
	Reduced-fat peanut butter	2 Tbsp	20 g	20 g	14 g	242
Snack 10 a.m.	Small apple	1	21 g	0	0	77
Lunch 12:30 p.m.	Chicken noodle soup	2 cups	14 g	8 g	14 g	180
	Side salad	2 cups	7 g	0	3 g	33
	Fat-free French dressing	1 Tbsp	5 g	0	0	21
Snack 3:30 p.m.	Cheddar and whole wheat crackers	4 crackers 4 oz cheese	16 g	12 g	28 g	264
Dinner 6 p.m.	Fast food hamburger	1 patty, 1 bun, condiments	47 g	27 g	25 g	531
	Side salad	2 cups	7 g	0	3 g	33
		Totals	189 g	69 g	97 g	1,645

Activity and Exercise

Activity	Time	Notes	Calories burned
Walking	20 min	1 mile	100
		Total	100

My Mood 1 = LOW, 10 = HIGH

Happiness	6	Anger	4	Hunger	2	Clarity	6
Stress	2	Energy	4	Health	8	Anxiety	1

HEALTH NOTES AND OBSERVATIONS: *Had lunch with a friend. Boss complimented me on marketing research report. Caught my favorite movie on television.*

MY DAILY HEALTH TRACKER

GOAL: ________________________ REWARD: ________________________

DATE: ____________ WEIGHT: ____________ HOURS OF SLEEP: ____________

Foods Eaten

Time	Food	Amount/Unit	Carbs	Fat	Protein	Calories
		Totals				

Activity and Exercise

Activity	Time	Notes	Calories burned
		Total	

My Mood 1 = LOW, 10 = HIGH

Happiness		Anger		Hunger		Clarity	
Stress		Energy		Health			

HEALTH NOTES AND OBSERVATIONS:

____

MY DAILY HEALTH TRACKER

GOAL: ___________________________ REWARD: ___________________________

DATE: _______________ WEIGHT: _______________ HOURS OF SLEEP: _______________

Foods Eaten

Time	Food	Amount/Unit	Carbs	Fat	Protein	Calories
		Totals				

Activity and Exercise

Activity	Time	Notes	Calories burned
		Total	

My Mood 1 = LOW, 10 = HIGH

Happiness		Anger		Hunger		Clarity	
Stress		Energy		Health			

HEALTH NOTES AND OBSERVATIONS: _______________________________________

____

MY **DAILY** HEALTH TRACKER

GOAL: ___________________________ REWARD: ___________________________

DATE: _______________ WEIGHT: _______________ HOURS OF SLEEP: _______________

Foods Eaten

Time	Food	Amount/Unit	Carbs	Fat	Protein	Calories
		Totals				

Activity and Exercise

Activity	Time	Notes	Calories burned
		Total	

My Mood 1 = LOW, 10 = HIGH

Happiness		Anger		Hunger		Clarity	
Stress		Energy		Health			

HEALTH NOTES AND OBSERVATIONS: ___________________________

____

MY DAILY HEALTH TRACKER

GOAL: ________________________ REWARD: ________________________

DATE: ____________ WEIGHT: ____________ HOURS OF SLEEP: ____________

Foods Eaten

Time	Food	Amount/Unit	Carbs	Fat	Protein	Calories
		Totals				

Activity and Exercise

Activity	Time	Notes	Calories burned
		Total	

My Mood 1 = LOW, 10 = HIGH

Happiness		Anger		Hunger		Clarity	
Stress		Energy		Health			

HEALTH NOTES AND OBSERVATIONS:

____

MY **DAILY** HEALTH TRACKER

GOAL: ___________________________   REWARD: ___________________________

DATE: _______________   WEIGHT: _______________   HOURS OF SLEEP: _______________

Foods Eaten

Time	Food	Amount/Unit	Carbs	Fat	Protein	Calories
		Totals				

Activity and Exercise

Activity	Time	Notes	Calories burned
		Total	

My Mood   1 = LOW, 10 = HIGH

Happiness		Anger		Hunger		Clarity	
Stress		Energy		Health			

HEALTH NOTES AND OBSERVATIONS:

____

MY DAILY HEALTH TRACKER

GOAL: _______________________   REWARD: _______________________

DATE: ____________   WEIGHT: ____________   HOURS OF SLEEP: ____________

Foods Eaten

Time	Food	Amount/Unit	Carbs	Fat	Protein	Calories
		Totals				

Activity and Exercise

Activity	Time	Notes	Calories burned
		Total	

My Mood   1 = LOW, 10 = HIGH

Happiness		Anger		Hunger		Clarity	
Stress		Energy		Health			

HEALTH NOTES AND OBSERVATIONS:

____

MY DAILY HEALTH TRACKER

GOAL: ________________________________ REWARD: ________________________________

DATE: ______________ WEIGHT: ______________ HOURS OF SLEEP: ______________

Foods Eaten

Time	Food	Amount/Unit	Carbs	Fat	Protein	Calories
		Totals				

Activity and Exercise

Activity	Time	Notes	Calories burned
		Total	

My Mood   1 = LOW, 10 = HIGH

Happiness		Anger		Hunger		Clarity	
Stress		Energy		Health			

HEALTH NOTES AND OBSERVATIONS: ________________________________

____

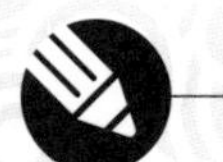 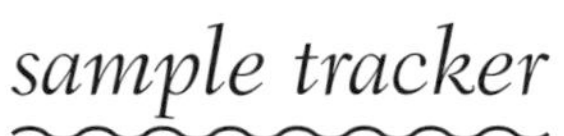

MY WEEKLY HEALTH TRACKER

You can also record your stats online at www.prevention.com/healthtrackers.

DATE: 2/6/11

WEEKLY GOALS	HOW DID I DO?	REWARD
Get more sleep	Mostly accomplished	Mani-pedi
Exercise 30 min/day	Missed 3 days	None

	Monday	Tuesday	Wednesday
Exercise?	Yes____ No__X__	Yes__X__ No____	Yes__X__ No____
Activity		Walk	Walk
Time		30 min	30 min
Weight	156 lbs	155 lbs	156 lbs
Hours of sleep	6	5	5
Food			
Breakfast	Pancakes, sm. apple, baby carrots & hummus	Yogurt & grapefruit	Protein shake
Lunch	Chicken salad & bagel	Salad	Portobello mushroom sandwich
Dinner	Fish and broccoli	Chicken, brown rice w. carrots	Pizza & salad
Snacks	Sm. apple, baby carrots & hummus	Sm. apple, cookies	Celery & hummus, cookies
Vitamins/meds	Multi	Multi	Multi
Describe mood	Irritated	Calm	Irritated
Joys	Had lunch with a friend	Told great joke at meeting, enjoyed chocolate snack	None I can think of
Stresses	Too much work	Too much work	Too much work; think I'm getting sick

83

NOTES: *Definitely felt crankier on days I got less sleep. Also harder to motivate myself to exercise then.*

Thursday	Friday	Saturday	Sunday
Yes___ No_X_	Yes_X_ No___	Yes_X_ No___	Yes___ No_X_
	Walk	Yoga	
	30 min	45 min	
157 lbs	157 lbs	156 lbs	156 lbs
8	8	6	9
Food			
Yogurt & grapefruit	Protein shake	Protein shake	Pancakes
Cold pizza & salad	Burger, no bun	Salad	Baked potato w. cheese
Chicken, mixed vegetables	Chinese chicken & broccoli	Fish and baked potato	Steak w. mushroom & squash
Sm. apple, cheese stick	Cheese stick, cookies	Chips, banana smoothie	Orange, cookies
Multi, ibuprofen	Multi	Multi	Multi, ibuprofen
Happy	Calm	Irritated	Happy
Coworker apologized, finished my project, impressed my boss	Stranger held door open for me, coworker complimented my new haircut	Mechanic bill was under $100	Slept in late, read in bed with breakfast
Car's making funny noises	Car's still making funny noises	Brought work home, late for yoga class	None

MY WEEKLY HEALTH TRACKER

You can also record your stats online at www.prevention.com/healthtrackers.

DATE: ___________________

WEEKLY GOALS	HOW DID I DO?	REWARD

	Monday	Tuesday	Wednesday
Exercise?			
Activity			
Time			
Weight			
Hours of sleep			
Food			
Breakfast			
Lunch			
Dinner			
Snacks			
Vitamins/meds			
Describe mood			
Joys			
Stresses			

NOTES:

Thursday	Friday	Saturday	Sunday
Food			

MY WEEKLY HEALTH TRACKER

You can also record your stats online at www.prevention.com/healthtrackers.

DATE: _______________________

WEEKLY GOALS	HOW DID I DO?	REWARD

	Monday	Tuesday	Wednesday
Exercise?			
Activity			
Time			
Weight			
Hours of sleep			
Food			
Breakfast			
Lunch			
Dinner			
Snacks			
Vitamins/meds			
Describe mood			
Joys			
Stresses			

NOTES:

Thursday	Friday	Saturday	Sunday
Food			

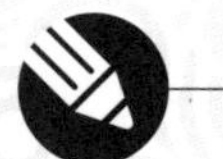

MY WEEKLY HEALTH TRACKER

You can also record your stats online at www.prevention.com/healthtrackers.

DATE: ___________________________

WEEKLY GOALS	HOW DID I DO?	REWARD

	Monday	Tuesday	Wednesday
Exercise?			
Activity			
Time			
Weight			
Hours of sleep			
Food			
Breakfast			
Lunch			
Dinner			
Snacks			
Vitamins/meds			
Describe mood			
Joys			
Stresses			

89

NOTES:

Thursday	Friday	Saturday	Sunday
Food			

my health journal

# MY WEEKLY HEALTH TRACKER

You can also record your stats online at www.prevention.com/healthtrackers.

DATE: ________________________

WEEKLY GOALS	HOW DID I DO?	REWARD

	Monday	Tuesday	Wednesday
Exercise?			
Activity			
Time			
Weight			
Hours of sleep			
Food			
Breakfast			
Lunch			
Dinner			
Snacks			
Vitamins/meds			
Describe mood			
Joys			
Stresses			

91

NOTES:

Thursday	Friday	Saturday	Sunday
Food			

my health journal

MY YEARLY HEALTH TRACKER

THE NEXT SEVERAL PAGES are designed to provide you with the space to track your vital health stats over a period of 5 years, but feel free to photocopy them to use after that if you choose. Some measures should be tracked frequently, once a month or more. Others are checked annually or every few years, depending on age. As a bonus, you'll be reminded about what tests might be due and how often you should be scheduling them. We've also given you some space to individualize with any additional tests your doctor may recommend.

YEAR: *2010*   AGE: *34*

Monthly Health Information (JANUARY THROUGH JUNE)

	January	February	March	April	May	June
Weight	*156*	*157*	*157*	*153*	*150*	*145*
BMI	27	27	27	27	26	25
BP			142			
			93			
Triglyceride level			192			
Cholesterol level total			48			
HDL/LDL			133			
Blood sugar (fasting blood glucose level)			80			
Waist circumference	37	37	37	37	36.5	36
Menstrual cycles	*14–20*	*13–20*	*14–19*	*15–20*	*15–21*	*13–19*
Doctors' visits			3			
Injuries/illnesses dates (see notes)	*22–27* *Cold*				*5–6* *Flu*	

NOTES: *Frustrating that after all this work to lose weight and improve my diet, my cholesterol levels haven't budged. But BP is down!*

Monthly Health Information (JULY THROUGH DECEMBER)

	July	August	September	October	November	December
Weight	143	143	140	144	142	147
BMI	25	25	24	25	25	25
BP	135					
	76					
Triglyceride level	180					
Cholesterol level total	48					
HDL/LDL	138					
Blood sugar (fasting blood glucose level)	78					
Waist circumference	36	36	35.5	36	36	36
Menstrual cycles	14–20	14–29	15–21	13–20	14–20	14–18
Doctors' visits	1		2			
Injuries/illnesses dates (see notes)			2 Ankle sprain	2–7 Cold		

Annual Health Information

Test	Needed	Date last done	Results	Next due
Physical exam	Annually	3/18/10	*BP & blood lipid profile a little high, lose 15 lbs*	3/2011
Clinical breast exam	Annually	3/20/10	*All clear*	3/2011
Dentist	Every 6 mo	3/20/10	*All clear*	9/18/10
Eye exam	Screen at 18, 32, as needed Every 2–4 yrs (40+)	*1/3/08*	*Vision is good, all clear*	*As needed*
Hearing test	Every 10 yrs	2/18/08	*All clear*	2018
Serum ferritin and transferrin saturation	Screen at 18, then monitor	3/18/10	*Good*	*N/A*
Pelvic exam/ Pap test/ STD tests	Every 3 yrs (50+) Annually (18+ or sexually active)	*3/20/10*	*All clear*	*3/2011*
Blood pressure	Every 2 yrs, or more often if elevated	*3/18/10*	*A little high*	*7/23/10*
Skin exam	Every 3 yrs (20+)	*3/18/10*		
Blood lipid profile	Every 5 yrs (20+), or more often if elevated	*3/18/10*	*Both cholesterol and triglycerides a little high*	*7/23/10*
Thyroid test (TSH)	Every 5 yrs (35+)	*N/A*		
Mammogram	Annually (40+)	*N/A*		
Colorectal cancer screening (Fecal Occult Blood Test)	Annually (50+)	*N/A*		
Bone density test	Annually (50+)	*N/A*		

This Year's Health Events:

PHYSICAL AND MENTAL HEALTH: DIAGNOSES AND DATES: *3/18/10 – Blood pressure, cholesterol, and triglycerides a little high. Doctor says I'm clinically overweight and need to lose 10–15 lbs to be in healthy BMI range.*

HOSPITAL VISITS: DATES AND OUTCOMES: *9/4/10 – Landed badly on ankle during volleyball game, went to ER. Just a bad sprain. Use ice and stay off of it for a few days.*

MAJOR ILLNESSES OR INJURIES AND DATES: *None*

PREGNANCIES/BIRTHS: *None*

OTHER MEDICAL EVENTS AND DATES: *None*

NOTES: *Stopped exercising as much when I hurt my ankle and immediately gained weight. Need to learn to adjust my diet better when that happens, but it's hard to deny myself treats when I'm in pain.*

MY YEARLY HEALTH TRACKER

YEAR: ___________________________   AGE: ___________________________

NOTES: ___________________________

____

____

____

Monthly Health Information (JANUARY THROUGH JUNE)

	January	February	March	April	May	June
Weight						
BMI						
BP						
Triglyceride level						
Cholesterol level total						
HDL/LDL						
Blood sugar (fasting blood glucose level)						
Waist circumference						
Menstrual cycles						
Doctors' visits						
Injuries/illnesses dates (see notes)						

NOTES:

Monthly Health Information (JULY THROUGH DECEMBER)

	July	August	September	October	November	December
Weight						
BMI						
BP						
Triglyceride level						
Cholesterol level total						
HDL/LDL						
Blood sugar (fasting blood glucose level)						
Waist circumference						
Menstrual cycles						
Doctors' visits						
Injuries/illnesses dates (see notes)						

my health journal

Annual Health Information

Test	Needed	Date last done	Results	Next due
Physical exam	Annually			
Clinical breast exam	Annually			
Dentist	Every 6 mo			
Eye exam	Screen at 18, 32, as needed Every 2–4 yrs (40+)			
Hearing test	Every 10 yrs			
Serum ferritin and transferrin saturation	Screen at 18, then monitor			
Pelvic exam/ Pap test/ STD tests	Every 3 yrs (50+) Annually (18+ or sexually active)			
Blood pressure	Every 2 yrs, or more often if elevated			
Skin exam	Every 3 yrs (20+)			
Blood lipid profile	Every 5 yrs (20+), or more often if elevated			
Thyroid test (TSH)	Every 5 yrs (35+)			
Mammogram	Annually (40+)			
Colorectal cancer screening (Fecal Occult Blood Test)	Annually (50+)			
Bone density test	Annually (50+)			

This Year's Health Events:

PHYSICAL AND MENTAL HEALTH: DIAGNOSES AND DATES:

HOSPITAL VISITS: DATES AND OUTCOMES:

MAJOR ILLNESSES OR INJURIES AND DATES:

PREGNANCIES/BIRTHS:

OTHER MEDICAL EVENTS AND DATES:

NOTES:

my health journal

 # MY YEARLY HEALTH TRACKER

YEAR: ________________________   AGE: ________________________

NOTES: ____

____

____

____

Monthly Health Information (JANUARY THROUGH JUNE)

	January	February	March	April	May	June
Weight						
BMI						
BP						
Triglyceride level						
Cholesterol level total						
HDL/LDL						
Blood sugar (fasting blood glucose level)						
Waist circumference						
Menstrual cycles						
Doctors' visits						
Injuries/illnesses dates (see notes)						

NOTES:

Monthly Health Information (JULY THROUGH DECEMBER)

	July	August	September	October	November	December
Weight						
BMI						
BP						
Triglyceride level						
Cholesterol level total						
HDL/LDL						
Blood sugar (fasting blood glucose level)						
Waist circumference						
Menstrual cycles						
Doctors' visits						
Injuries/illnesses dates (see notes)						

my health journal

Annual Health Information

Test	Needed	Date last done	Results	Next due
Physical exam	Annually			
Clinical breast exam	Annually			
Dentist	Every 6 mo			
Eye exam	Screen at 18, 32, as needed Every 2–4 yrs (40+)			
Hearing test	Every 10 yrs			
Serum ferritin and transferrin saturation	Screen at 18, then monitor			
Pelvic exam/ Pap test/ STD tests	Every 3 yrs (50+) Annually (18+ or sexually active)			
Blood pressure	Every 2 yrs, or more often if elevated			
Skin exam	Every 3 yrs (20+)			
Blood lipid profile	Every 5 yrs (20+), or more often if elevated			
Thyroid test (TSH)	Every 5 yrs (35+)			
Mammogram	Annually (40+)			
Colorectal cancer screening (Fecal Occult Blood Test)	Annually (50+)			
Bone density test	Annually (50+)			

This Year's Health Events:

PHYSICAL AND MENTAL HEALTH: DIAGNOSES AND DATES:

HOSPITAL VISITS: DATES AND OUTCOMES:

MAJOR ILLNESSES OR INJURIES AND DATES:

PREGNANCIES/BIRTHS:

OTHER MEDICAL EVENTS AND DATES:

NOTES:

my health journal

MY YEARLY HEALTH TRACKER

YEAR: ___________________________   AGE: ___________________________

NOTES: ___________________________

____

____

____

Monthly Health Information (JANUARY THROUGH JUNE)

	January	February	March	April	May	June
Weight						
BMI						
BP						
Triglyceride level						
Cholesterol level total						
HDL/LDL						
Blood sugar (fasting blood glucose level)						
Waist circumference						
Menstrual cycles						
Doctors' visits						
Injuries/illnesses dates (see notes)						

NOTES:

____

____

____

Monthly Health Information (JULY THROUGH DECEMBER)

	July	August	September	October	November	December
Weight						
BMI						
BP						
Triglyceride level						
Cholesterol level total						
HDL/LDL						
Blood sugar (fasting blood glucose level)						
Waist circumference						
Menstrual cycles						
Doctors' visits						
Injuries/illnesses dates (see notes)						

Annual Health Information

Test	Needed	Date last done	Results	Next due
Physical exam	Annually			
Clinical breast exam	Annually			
Dentist	Every 6 mo			
Eye exam	Screen at 18, 32, as needed Every 2–4 yrs (40+)			
Hearing test	Every 10 yrs			
Serum ferritin and transferrin saturation	Screen at 18, then monitor			
Pelvic exam/ Pap test/ STD tests	Every 3 yrs (50+) Annually (18+ or sexually active)			
Blood pressure	Every 2 yrs, or more often if elevated			
Skin exam	Every 3 yrs (20+)			
Blood lipid profile	Every 5 yrs (20+), or more often if elevated			
Thyroid test (TSH)	Every 5 yrs (35+)			
Mammogram	Annually (40+)			
Colorectal cancer screening (Fecal Occult Blood Test)	Annually (50+)			
Bone density test	Annually (50+)			

This Year's Health Events:

PHYSICAL AND MENTAL HEALTH: DIAGNOSES AND DATES:

HOSPITAL VISITS: DATES AND OUTCOMES:

MAJOR ILLNESSES OR INJURIES AND DATES:

PREGNANCIES/BIRTHS:

OTHER MEDICAL EVENTS AND DATES:

NOTES:

my health journal

MY YEARLY HEALTH TRACKER

YEAR: ________________________   AGE: ________________________

NOTES: ____

____

____

____

Monthly Health Information (JANUARY THROUGH JUNE)

	January	February	March	April	May	June
Weight						
BMI						
BP						
Triglyceride level						
Cholesterol level total						
HDL/LDL						
Blood sugar (fasting blood glucose level)						
Waist circumference						
Menstrual cycles						
Doctors' visits						
Injuries/illnesses dates (see notes)						

NOTES:

____

____

____

Monthly Health Information (JULY THROUGH DECEMBER)

	July	August	September	October	November	December
Weight						
BMI						
BP						
Triglyceride level						
Cholesterol level total						
HDL/LDL						
Blood sugar (fasting blood glucose level)						
Waist circumference						
Menstrual cycles						
Doctors' visits						
Injuries/illnesses dates (see notes)						

my health journal

Annual Health Information

Test	Needed	Date last done	Results	Next due
Physical exam	Annually			
Clinical breast exam	Annually			
Dentist	Every 6 mo			
Eye exam	Screen at 18, 32, as needed Every 2–4 yrs (40+)			
Hearing test	Every 10 yrs			
Serum ferritin and transferrin saturation	Screen at 18, then monitor			
Pelvic exam/ Pap test/ STD tests	Every 3 yrs (50+) Annually (18+ or sexually active)			
Blood pressure	Every 2 yrs, or more often if elevated			
Skin exam	Every 3 yrs (20+)			
Blood lipid profile	Every 5 yrs (20+), or more often if elevated			
Thyroid test (TSH)	Every 5 yrs (35+)			
Mammogram	Annually (40+)			
Colorectal cancer screening (Fecal Occult Blood Test)	Annually (50+)			
Bone density test	Annually (50+)			

This Year's Health Events:

PHYSICAL AND MENTAL HEALTH: DIAGNOSES AND DATES:

HOSPITAL VISITS: DATES AND OUTCOMES:

MAJOR ILLNESSES OR INJURIES AND DATES:

PREGNANCIES/BIRTHS:

OTHER MEDICAL EVENTS AND DATES:

NOTES:

MY YEARLY HEALTH TRACKER

YEAR: ___________________________   AGE: ___________________________

NOTES: ___________________________

____

____

____

Monthly Health Information (JANUARY THROUGH JUNE)

	January	February	March	April	May	June
Weight						
BMI						
BP						
Triglyceride level						
Cholesterol level total						
HDL/LDL						
Blood sugar (fasting blood glucose level)						
Waist circumference						
Menstrual cycles						
Doctors' visits						
Injuries/illnesses dates (see notes)						

NOTES:

____

____

____

____

Monthly Health Information (JULY THROUGH DECEMBER)

	July	August	September	October	November	December
Weight						
BMI						
BP						
Triglyceride level						
Cholesterol level total						
HDL/LDL						
Blood sugar (fasting blood glucose level)						
Waist circumference						
Menstrual cycles						
Doctors' visits						
Injuries/illnesses dates (see notes)						

Annual Health Information

Test	Needed	Date last done	Results	Next due
Physical exam	Annually			
Clinical breast exam	Annually			
Dentist	Every 6 mo			
Eye exam	Screen at 18, 32, as needed Every 2–4 yrs (40+)			
Hearing test	Every 10 yrs			
Serum ferritin and transferrin saturation	Screen at 18, then monitor			
Pelvic exam/ Pap test/ STD tests	Every 3 yrs (50+) Annually (18+ or sexually active)			
Blood pressure	Every 2 yrs, or more often if elevated			
Skin exam	Every 3 yrs (20+)			
Blood lipid profile	Every 5 yrs (20+), or more often if elevated			
Thyroid test (TSH)	Every 5 yrs (35+)			
Mammogram	Annually (40+)			
Colorectal cancer screening (Fecal Occult Blood Test)	Annually (50+)			
Bone density test	Annually (50+)			

This Year's Health Events:

PHYSICAL AND MENTAL HEALTH: DIAGNOSES AND DATES:

HOSPITAL VISITS: DATES AND OUTCOMES:

MAJOR ILLNESSES OR INJURIES AND DATES:

PREGNANCIES/BIRTHS:

OTHER MEDICAL EVENTS AND DATES:

NOTES:

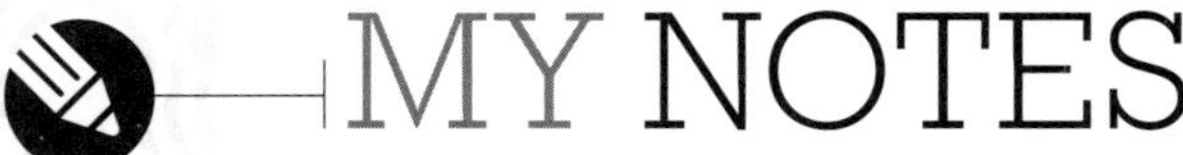

MY NOTES

THOUGH YOU'LL FIND A WEALTH of charts designed for tracking all sorts of health measures and information, as well as checklists and self-care lists, you'll occasionally want to create some lists of your own, such as bad habits you want to break, new healthy foods you want to incorporate into your diet, or even family members you've been meaning to talk to about their health history. Here's some room to do that or to write any other notes you want to keep handy with the rest of your information.

IN CASE OF **EMERGENCY**

TEAR THIS SHEET OUT and place it somewhere easily visible, such as on your refrigerator or a family bulletin board. If you have children, you may want to review these potentially dangerous symptoms so that they can call 911 for you in case of an emergency.

→ CALL 911 IMMEDIATELY IF YOU HAVE:

- ☐ **CHEST PAIN**, especially if it's accompanied by tightness that spreads to your arms, back, neck, or jaw; breathlessness; nausea; light-headedness; or a cold sweat. Important note: Women having a heart attack may experience more discomfort, pressure, or tightness in their chests and the other above-mentioned symptoms than actual chest pain.

- ☐ **SHORTNESS OF BREATH**, especially if it's accompanied by confusion, light-headedness, hives, heart palpitations, and nausea

- ☐ **NUMBNESS OR WEAKNESS IN YOUR FACE**, arm, or leg, especially if it's only on one side of your body

- ☐ **SUDDEN LOSS OF ABILITIES SUCH AS WALKING**, speaking, seeing clearly, thinking, or understanding what other people are saying

- ☐ **SUDDEN AND SEVERE HEADACHES**, especially if you've just suffered a head injury or if the headache is accompanied by a stiff neck, fever, rash, difficulty concentrating, or seizures

- ☐ **UNCONTROLLABLE BLEEDING**. If you have a bloody nose that just won't stop or are bleeding from the ears, vomiting blood, or have a minor injury that won't clot

- ☐ **LOSS OF CONSCIOUSNESS**, especially if accompanied by confusion; deep, rapid breathing; hot, dry, flushed red skin; or seizures

→ CALL YOUR DOCTOR IMMEDIATELY IF YOU HAVE:

- ☐ **BLOODY STOOL**. Bloody stool may appear black and tarry or more burgundy or bright red depending on where it's coming from. If accompanied by weakness, call 911.

- ☐ **UNUSUAL HEADACHES**, especially if you've suffered a head injury in the past or if the headache is accompanied by a stiff neck, fever, rash, or difficulty concentrating

- ☐ **LUMPS OR THICKENED SPOTS**

- ☐ **BLEEDING OR UNUSUAL DISCHARGE** such as bloody phlegm (material you cough up), blood in the urine, blood or discharge from the nipple, bloody vomit, or unusual vaginal bleeding

- ☐ **THOUGHTS ABOUT HURTING YOURSELF OR SOMEONE ELSE**

- ☐ **HEARING VOICES OR SEEING THINGS**

- ☐ **INTENSE, UNEXPLAINABLE FEAR**, especially if accompanied by sweating, pounding heart, shortness of breath, and shaking